European Practice in Gynaecology and Obstetrics

Invasive carcinoma of the cervix

European Practice in Gynaecology and Obstetrics

Invasive carcinoma of the cervix

Volume Editor
G. Body (France)

P. Benedetti Panici (Italy)
G. Body (France)
P. Bösze (Hungary)
F. Fétissof (France)
S. Fotiou (Greece)
T. Mould (UK)
A. Norström (Sweden)

C. De Oliviera (Portugal)
D. Querleu (France)
A. Sasco (France)
M. Shafi (UK)
E. Van Limbergen (Belgium)
R. Winter (Austria)
J. Xercavins (Spain)

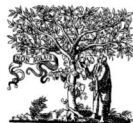
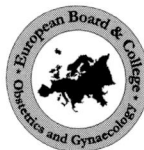

ELSEVIER

Editions Scientifiques et Médicales Elsevier, 23, rue Linois, 75724 Paris cedex 15
Member of Elsevier Science
http://www.emc.tm.fr - http://www.elsevier.fr

Printed in France by Jouve, 18, rue Saint-Denis, 75001 Paris
N° 303345S - Dépôt légal : Janvier 2002 - ISBN : 2-84299-306-3

Invasive carcinoma of the cervix

Contributing authors

A. Alonso (France)
M. Amoroso (Italy)
P. Benedetti Panici (Italy)
G. Body (France)
P. Bösze (Hungary)
P. Bougnoux
M. Congiu (Italy)
G. Cutillo (Italy)
F. Diallo-Diabaté (France)
F. Fétissof (France)
S. Fotiou (Greece)
A. Gil-Moreno (Spain)

C. Haie-Meder (France)
J. Jordan (UK)
J. Lansac (France)
E. Leblanc (France)
O. Le Floch (France)
F. Maneschi (Italy)
F. Mota (Portugal)
T. Mould (UK)
A. Norström (Sweden)
C. De Oliveira (Portugal)
I. Palaia (Italy)
F. Perrotin (France)

D. Querleu (France)
T. Rådberg (Sweden)
A. Rodolakis (Greece)
A. Sasco (France)
M. Shafi (UK)
J. Shepherd (UK)
K. Tamussino (Austria)
E. Van Limbergen (Belgium)
R. Winter (Austria)
J. Xercavins (Spain)

Scientific Committee

J. Lansac (France)
Chairman

J. Amy (Belgium), P. Bösze (Hungary), M. Cabero Roura (Spain), W. Dunlop (UK),
A. Goverde (Netherlands), I. Milsom (Sweden), F. Nunes (Portugal), K. Schneider (Germany),
B. Tarlatzis (Greece), V. Unzeiting (Czech Republic)

Editor in Chief: Caroline Chaine, M.D.

Editions Scientifiques et Médicales Elsevier
23, rue Linois
75724 Paris Cedex 15

c.chaine@elsevier.fr

Please send all correspondence to Dr. Chaine at the above address.

Table of Contents

Preface

Why this collection on "European Practice in Gynaecology and Obstetrics"?

The Europe Union is progressing.
Under the auspices of the European Board and College of Obstetrics and Gynaecology (EBCOG), recommendations have been published and accepted by the European Union of Medical Specialists (UEMS) in order to standardise the training of gynaecologists and obstetricians to ensure quality care and facilitate the exchange of physicians in European countries.
It was deemed that a series of books covering obstetrical and gynaecological practice was needed to provide up-to-date information for post-graduate students and the continuing education of specialists.
A common EBCOG and EAGO scientific committee is responsible for the contents of the collection. For each topic, this committee has selected the volume editor and the contributing authors, specialists throughout Europe known for their expertise in their fields. Each chapter is reviewed by external referees to assess the scientific quality of its contents and the evidence-based recommendations.
The authors describe the various types of management used in European practice, as well as the published results. They present those treatments for which a consensus exists; when there is no consensus, they discuss the key elements of the controversy.
In each book, the reader will find a review of the basic science, recent concepts in physiopathology, clinical aspects, treatment and unresolved problems or controversies, as well as the major recent references. A final section provides multiple choice questions covering each chapter.
We would like our readers to give us their opinions on these books so that we can continue to make this collection a useful tool for students and practising specialists alike.

Professor Jacques Lansac, MD, FRCOG
Chairman of the Scientific Committee

Introduction

At the beginning of the third millennium, what does carcinoma of the cervix uteri have in common with the disease in the 1970s and 1980s? Not much, really!

First of all, the epidemiology is no longer quite the same. In developed countries, cervical cancers are no longer the leading type of gynaecological cancer, but are now second to endometrial cancers. The incidence of carcinoma of the cervix is in sharp decline due to early screening and treatment of pre-invasive cancers. According to the "Annual Report on the Results of Treatment in Gynaecological Cancer", published in 1998 in the *Journal of Epidemiology and Biostatistics*, the number of cervical cancers during the period 1973-75 was 34,178 as compared to 12,153 for the period 1990-92. At the same time, the prognosis has improved, with a five year survival rate that has increased from 55.7% to 65.4%.

At present, MRI and laparoscopy have a very important role in the evaluation of the locoregional extension of the disease. Clinical examination must still be performed in all cases, as staging of cervical cancer is based on clinical evaluation alone. However, its reliability has been improved due to the progress made in imaging techniques, in particular magnetic resonance imaging (MRI).

The contributions of MRI are manyfold. It allows precise measurement of the volume of a tumour and analysis of its possible extension towards the corpus uteri. It also permits evaluation of parametrial spreading with an accuracy rate slightly higher than that of clinical examination (around 90%), of vesical and rectal spreading in late stage cancers not pertaining to surgery, and of nodal spreading with nearly 90% accuracy. Together with the clinical examination, MRI also helps evaluate tumour response during external radiotherapy, and at end of treatment, after uterovaginal curietherapy, in deciding whether or not to perform additional surgery.

The introduction of coelioscopy as a diagnostic tool allows highly accurate nodular evaluation. A complete curettage (pelvic and lumboaortic) prior to any therapeutic choice is a new approach, which basically indicates surgery for cancers with a good prognosis (pN0) and radiotherapy with or without associated chemotherapy (depending on tumour volume and nodular status) for all other cases.

All of these preoperative explorations now permit precise evaluation of the locoregional spread of the disease and of the main prognosis factors upon which depend the increasingly specific therapeutic indications.

New therapeutic means have significantly transformed the management of cervical cancers, especially for stages I and II. Two examples among the most meaningful are briefly presented here.

Today, the discovery of a cervical cancer no longer means loss of fertility, at least in early stage cancers, since D. Dargent in France devised the enlarged trachelectomy. This comprises a cervicectomy with colpectomy of the upper third of the vagina and ablation of the proximal part of the cardinal ligaments, associated with a coelioscopic interiliac lymphadenectomy. However, the preservation of fertility can only be envisaged for specific indications: cancer size ≤ 2 cm, tumours with endocervical spreading allowing a sufficient margin, absence of nodular invasion, and of course, the patient's desire to be pregnant. The results are promising in oncological terms and permit a reasonable probability of pregnancy (from 19 to 37% depending on the series); however, they do include relatively high risks of late abortion.

As concerns locally advanced cervical cancers (stage IB ≥ 4 cm, without lumboaortic nodular spreading), their poor prognosis has been significantly modified by the first very encouraging results published in 1999 by Keys (GOG study) and Morris (RTOG study) regarding concomitant radio-chemotherapy. These results show a reduced relative lethal risk of approximately 50% in the concomitant radiotherapy-chemotherapy group compared to the radiotherapy only group; this benefit is due more to an improvement of the pelvic control rather than of the distant control. This inroad raises new questions, among others the place of surgery after such an association because of increased morbidity, particularly at the urinary level.

Finally, with what we know today, how can we imagine tomorrow's responsibilities in treating cervical cancers? Their screening and diagnosis are still a major concern today and will remain so in the future, but one can surmise that they will increasingly be performed by highly specialised teams. Major laparoscopic pelvic and lumboaortic curettage can only be carried out by experienced gynaecologists or oncological surgeons; in the same way, radiotherapy with concomitant chemotherapy imposes close, complementary collaboration between the radiotherapist, the chemotherapist and, if necessary, the surgeon who will have to perform a more difficult surgical act, with higher morbidity. Obviously, this increased technicity combined with the decreasing number of cervical cancers to be treated will render incompatible the diversification of the physician's experience, on the one hand, and the demands of the new therapeutic methods, on the other.

The following pages have been written by European specialists in this pathology, from Austria, England, France, Greece, Hungary, Italy, Portugal, Spain, and Sweden. Their articles summarise their teams' experience and their personal opinions. I would like to make a comparison with the construction of Europe, where national specificity is increasingly put to the service of the Community. In the case of cervical cancer, the progress made now leads to the best treatment choice or the best therapeutic sequence, but also to the best adaptation to each particular case, leaving behind the debates between different schools of thought, especially between surgery and radiotherapy, which sometimes prevailed in the past. The reader, for his part, will be the greatest beneficiary and will find in this book the current state of knowledge in a field of gynaecological oncology which has changed greatly over the past twenty years.

Professor Gilles Body
Volume Editor

G Body, Professor, Service de Gynécologie Obstétrique C, Hôpital Bretonneau, 2, boulevard Tonnellé, 37044 Tours, France.

Chapter 1

New concepts in epidemiology of cervical carcinoma

Annie J Sasco

AJ Sasco, M.D., Dr P.H., Chief, Unit of Epidemiology for Cancer Prevention, International Agency for Research on Cancer, Director of Research, Institut National de la Santé et de la Recherche Médicale, 150 cours Albert Thomas, 69008 Lyon, France.

New concepts in epidemiology of cervical carcinoma

AJ Sasco

Abstract. – **Descriptive epidemiology:** *In terms of world mortality, cervical carcinoma ranks fifth among cancers in women and third in terms of incidence. Whereas incidence rates (standardised to the age structure of the world population) vary from a minimum of 2.6 new cases per 100,000 woman-years in China to a maximum of 67.2 in Africans from Harare, Zimbabwe, European rates vary from 3.4 to 20.6, with most rates being between 7 and 12. Secular analysis indicates a general downward trend.*
Aetiologic epidemiology: *Traditional risk factors for cervical cancer have been linked to sexual behaviour (age at first intercourse, multiple partners), reproductive life (high number of pregnancies, use of oral contraceptives), socio-economic factors (low social class and education, ethnicity) and, more recently, tobacco. Current aetiology focuses on human papilloma viruses (HPV), of which several strains have been recognised as carcinogenic. This opens the way to potential preventive strategies based on immunisation.*

Keywords: mortality, risk factor, sexual life, human papilloma virus, tobacco, socio-economic condition.

Introduction

Cervical carcinoma may qualify as one of the cancers for which the acquisition of knowledge about aetiology has been the most drastic during the last 20 years. From an ill-defined array of mostly behavioural and social determinants to the demonstration of the causative role of a family of viruses, the new data have led to a better understanding of the natural history of the disease – from successful screening strategies with the use of the Papanicolaou smear (unfortunately, only currently practical in the developed world) to the entertainment of the possibility of primary prevention through viral immunisation. Although still at a pre-experimental stage, vaccines could be the most efficient weapons in combating the epidemic of this disease in the developing world. Therefore, from the point of view of scientific knowledge, cancer of the uterine cervix is in epidemiologic transition: from a vaguely aetiologically-defined condition to a perfectly-characterised one; from a clinical condition exclusively treated at the invasive stage by a surgical approach to the challenge of monitoring a chronic viral infection; and finally and most importantly, from a public health point of view, from a disease adequately screened in populations at low-to-moderate risk, to the hope of preventing the occurrence of invasion through viral immunisation in high-risk groups.

Descriptive epidemiology

The incidence and mortality of the disease may always be described along at least two axes: place and time.

■ Current world mortality and incidence

Current world mortality

The most recent estimate of total mortality linked to cervical cancer in the world is 237,000 deaths for the year 1998, corresponding to 0.9% of total female mortality. Most of these deaths occur in countries with a low-to-medium income, with 220,000 deaths (0.5%), whereas countries with a high income account only for 17,000 deaths, or 0.2% of female mortality [43].

Yet, mortality alone provides relatively poor information about the total disease burden, because, on one hand, cervical cancer is far from always being fatal, and on the other hand, many cases are totally passed over due to inaccuracy in death certification. The distinction between cervix and corpus uteri is not systematically made, even in some European countries, leading to uncertainties about the precise number of deaths attributable to cervical cancer. For the developing world, the problem is much more complex and current figures concerning the total disease burden are in large part estimated, rather than actual, counts [43].

Altogether, cancer of the uterine cervix ranks fifth for cancer mortality in women, following breast, lung, stomach and colorectal cancers [42, 43].

Current world incidence

An estimate of the total number of incident cases of cervical carcinoma in the world is 430,000 for the year 1997. Most occur in the developing world with 340,000 cases, in contrast to 90,000 in the developed nations. This corresponds to an estimated prevalence world-wide of 3,955,000 women with cervical cancer [42].

By far the most common cancer among women world-wide is breast cancer, representing in terms of incidence and for 1990, 21% of all cancer cases in women. Following breast cancer, we find in decreasing order of frequency cancer of the colorectum (10.1%), with cancer of the cervix in third position (9.8%). The ranking differs between developed and developing countries. Whereas it ranks second in the latter after breast cancer, it only comes seventh in the former, following breast, colorectum, lung, stomach, corpus uteri and ovary cancers [32].

The best available data on incidence comes from population-based cancer registries. These now exist in all continents and cover geographically and racially diverse populations. They provide knowledge on the source population, in terms of sex and age distribution, and exhaustive data collection of all new cancer cases occurring in a geographically defined, resident population. The IARC publication, Cancer Incidence In Five Continents, puts together this information at the world level [33]. The highest incidence rate (age-standardised to the structure of the world population) is found for African women in Harare, Zimbabwe, with 67.2 new cases per 100,000 woman-years (wy). Rates above 30 per 100,000 wy are encountered in another cancer registry in Africa, with 40.8 in Kyadondo, Uganda, and in several Central and South American registries, such as Concordia, Argentina (32.0); Belem, (64.8) and Goiania (37.1), Brazil; Cali, Columbia (34.4); Quito, Ecuador (31.7); Trujillo, Peru (53.5). The only other cancer registries with a rate above 30 are for the Maori population in New Zealand at 32.2, and Madras, India (38.9).

In North America, rates range from 4.1 for the Japanese population of Los Angeles, USA, to 17.9 for Hispanic white women, also of Los Angeles. Most rates are around 7 to 12 new cases per 100,000 wy. The fact that both the lowest and highest rates for the entire North American continent are found in the same cancer registry, but for different racial groups, clearly indicates the importance of ethnicity as a risk factor for cervical cancer. In United States cancer registries which present data separately for each ethnic group, Hispanics tend to have the highest rates, followed by the black population. In contrast, the rates for Asians are usually lower than those of the white population.

As suggested by the above figures concerning migrants, or their descendants, to the New World, the rates of most Asian populations are quite low. This applies to China, which has the lowest world recorded rate of cervical cancer at 2.6 per 100,000 wy in Qidong, as well as other rates below five (Shanghai at 3.3 and Tianjin at 4.4). In Japan, rates vary from 5.5 in Yamagata to 12.6 in Hiroshima. Rates in Thailand and India are higher, from 15.7 in Karunagappally, India to 38.9 in Madras, India.

In Oceania, most of the rates, with the exception of some migrant groups to Hawaii, USA, are around 10 per 100,000. The highest rates are recorded in French Polynesia at 27.7 and for the Maori of New Zealand at 32.2.

European rates will be described below.

Another way of presenting incidence, often more intuitive to clinicians than age-standardised incidence rates, is to give cumulative incidence. This represents the probability of developing the disease over a life-span, or, more often, from age 0 to 74 years, to avoid errors due to differential reporting of diagnosis in the most elderly sector of the population. This measure is then simply expressed as a percentage. For cervical cancer, cumulative incidence varies from 0.3% in Qidong, China to 6.9% for Belem, Brazil: a 23-fold difference. Again, high values are found in Central and South America, but also in India. In contrast, North American and European values are intermediary.

■ Current European mortality and incidence

Detailed data on cancer are available for all countries, but are particularly rich for the member states of the European Union [17].

Current European mortality

For the year 1995, the age-standardised mortality rate in the European Union as a whole was 3.23 deaths per 100,000 wy. The lowest rate was recorded in Luxembourg at 0.22 per 100,000 and the highest in Denmark at 4.73. Two countries had rates lower than 1 per 100 000, Luxembourg and Finland (0.92). Six countries had rates between 1 and 3: 1.82 for the Netherlands, 2.04 for Greece, 2.50 for Sweden, 2.56 for Spain, 2.65 for Italy and 2.95 for Belgium. Finally, seven countries were above 3: 3.43 for France, 3.64 for the United Kingdom and Ireland, 3.80 for Germany, 4.56 for Portugal, 4.66 for Austria and 4.73 for Denmark.

Overall, mortality rates for cervical cancer in the European Union are moderate. Rates in other European countries, and in particular in the former Eastern block, are higher.

Current European incidence

Again, detailed information may be found for countries of the European Union [17].

In the European Union as a whole and for 1995, the age-standardised rate was 9.87 new cases per 100,000 wy. The lowest rate was at 2.66 in Luxembourg. The highest rate was recorded for Portugal at 14.74. Rates below five were found for two countries, Luxembourg and Finland, the latter being at 4.43. Rates between five and ten concerned seven countries: 6.29 for the Netherlands, 6.87 for Spain, 7.25 for Greece, 7.26 for Sweden, 7.67 for Ireland, 8.00 for Belgium and 9.00 for Italy. Finally, six countries had rates above 10: 10.02 for France, 10.74 for the United Kingdom, 12.08 for Germany, 12.22 for Austria, 13.17 for Denmark and 14.74 for Portugal [17].

Among other European countries not belonging to the European Union, patterns differ according to place. Switzerland had rates below ten, from 5.4 in Basle to 9.8 in Graubunden. Similarly, Iceland was at 8.0. Countries of the previous Eastern block had much higher rates, all above 10 and several above 15, with the exception of Latvia at 9.5. Rates of 16.4 in the Czech Republic, between 15.2 (in Warsaw) and 21.8 in lower Silesia in Poland, or 17.7 in Vojvodina, Yugoslavia, were described [33].

Figures of prevalence representing an estimation of the number of women currently being and having been, in a given period, diagnosed with cervical cancer have been produced for member states of the European Union. Altogether, the European Union counts 99,801 cases for 5-year prevalence, whereas the 1- and 3-year estimates are at 23,126 and 66,094, respectively [17]. Although several assumptions and uncertainties are embodied in these figures, they provide some information of interest to care givers, be they medically or more socially oriented.

■ Time trends in mortality, incidence and survival

Descriptive epidemiology of cancer does not remain static over time. Changes in incidence are the most likely to provide the basis for aetiological clues, but may also yield information on screening activities. In contrast, changes in mortality reflect both the evolution of incidence and modification of treatment. Survival and its secular trend yield the most direct way of evaluating treatment effectiveness.

Time trends in mortality

The mortality data for cervical cancer are unfortunately not very informative, given the large numbers of deaths certified as "uterus, not otherwise specified", and not specifically assigned either to the cervix or corpus uteri. As already stated above, this remains a problem even for current statistics, but is an even more serious impediment to the evaluation of trends over time, since large differences between countries in the allocation of deaths to the specific parts of the uterus, as well as a general decline in under-certification of deaths as due to cervical cancer, may bias the assessment of trends in mortality [11]. The general pattern is one of decreasing mortality rates in most countries of the world, the magnitude varying depending on populations. In the Americas, percentage changes per five-year periods between 1975 and 1988 were on the order of 5 to 15% with, in most places, relatively modest differences according to age groups. Similar effects were seen for Asia and Oceania, although some countries, such as Mauritius, reported increases instead.

Whether or not they belong to the European Community, most countries in Europe experienced decreases between less than 10% and up to more than 35% per five-year periods. Yet there were exceptions to this general pattern, for example in Spain, the United Kingdom, Czechoslovakia and Hungary, where increases were noted. When looking more carefully at these changes, it is worth noting that the younger age group, 30 to 44 years of age, has experienced particularly large increases, on the order of 20 to 30% in Spain, Greece, the United Kingdom as well as Czechoslovakia and Hungary. This is particularly noteworthy as the quality of death certification data is likely to be least problematic for younger women. In addition, most of the deaths are likely to be due to cervical cancer, due to the rarity of cancer of the corpus uteri in this age group. If reallocation of deaths coded as "uterus, not otherwise specified" is done using identical percentages for all age groups, this will lead to an under-estimation of cervical cancer in young women. In contrast, an observed increase in mortality may be partly ascribed to better registration and a corresponding decrease in the number of deaths attributed to "uterus, not otherwise specified" [11].

Time trends in incidence

Data on incidence do not suffer many of the limitations ascribed to mortality data. On a world scale and in terms of ranking by decreasing order of absolute number of incident cases, cervical cancer is losing some of its importance, in the developing world in particular. Estimations have been carried out at the world level since 1980. The cervix was the leading cancer site for women in less developed regions of the world up to the year 1990 [30, 31]. Since 1990, it is remarkable to note that in both developed and less developed regions, cervical cancer now ranks after breast cancer for women [32]. From 344,000 cervical and 298,000 breast cancers for the less developed countries in 1985 [31], we went to 286,012 cervical and 323,101 breast cancers in 1990 [32], showing in parallel a decrease in cervical cancer and an increase in breast cancer. Therefore, cervical cancer is no longer the leading female cancer, as it was for so long in the poorer countries. The increase of breast cancer is a challenge to all clinicians and researchers wherever they practice.

A more detailed analysis may be conducted using population-based cancer registries. Decreases are seen in most places and are quite large, up to a 30 to 40% decrease per five-year period. In Asia and Oceania, this decrease is seen for most Asian populations, except the Chinese and Malays in Singapore. The rate of decline is less marked in India but very rapid in China where it is greater than 40% per five-year period in Shanghai.

In the Americas, with the exception of Cuba, decreases are also seen, albeit of a somewhat smaller magnitude. In Canada and the United States, declines were steady for a while but then reached a plateau, and may even be replaced by an increase in the younger age groups.

In Europe, the general trend is a steep decline, except in Spain and the United Kingdom. Among non-member states of the European Union, the decline is also particularly marked in Switzerland and Slovenia. Among member states, one should single out the United Kingdom, where increases are seen, particularly in young women, and are particularly marked in Birmingham and Scotland. Almost all age groups, with the possible exception of the eldest, are affected by an increase in Spain [11].

Explanations offered for the downward trend in incidence include coverage of the population by well-organised cancer screening programmes [10, 19] and access to medical care with better treatment [36]. In contrast, the increases especially seen in the younger age groups are more difficult to explain. Less optimal screening in young women has been advanced as an explanation, as well as real increases in incidence due to modifications both of sexual activity and cancer prevention practices [11].

Part of the reason for an unclear picture is the grouping of different histological types of cancer in population-based statistics. Of particular note in this respect is the increase in invasive adenocarcinoma of the cervix [15]. This cancer seen in young women is more difficult to discover with routine screening by Pap test and may have a poorer survival rate [1, 38]. Such a distinction could help in better understanding trends and also in elucidating aetiology. It should be noted that even in countries where increases were seen in the 80s and early 90s, more recent data may be reassuring [40]. Yet studies of pre-cancerous lesions seem to indicate the need to continue targeted screening in some young women [6].

Time trends in survival

Survival from cervical cancer depends on the stage of the disease at diagnosis. Surgery is by far the most important approach. In general, in the early stages the results are excellent.

Five-year, age-standardised relative survivals in Europe are consistently greater than 50%. For Europe as a whole and for the 1985-89 diagnosis period, the five-year survival rate is 61.8%, varying from 51.0% in Poland to 84.7% in Iceland. Survival is inversely related to age, with figures of 75% for 15-44 year-olds, 63% for 45-54, 60% for 55-64, 52% for 65-74 and only 36% for women older than 75 [2]. Compared to preceding periods [3] survival demonstrates some slight improvement, from 59% to 62%, also seen in most age groups.

Overall, survival is good and improving, although the observed changes are not drastic.

Aetiologic epidemiology

It has long been known that cervical cancer is linked to sexual activity, but the demonstration of the role of a sexually-transmitted virus, the human papilloma virus (HPV), is more recent.

- ### Classical risk factors: sexual and reproductive life, socio-economic conditions

It was already noted in past centuries that cervical cancer was extremely rare among nuns, and in contrast, strongly associated with sexual activity. Two factors are important:

the age at first intercourse and the number of sexual partners. The younger a woman is when she first has sexual intercourse, the higher her risk of subsequent cervical cancer [5]. Yet, even more important for establishing the risk, and even more strongly in favour of sexual transmission of an infectious agent, is the number of sexual partners [23]. In fact, at least in some countries, the number of sexual partners of the male is more important than the number of partners of the woman herself [35]. This effect of the man's partners is particularly clear when looking at women who have only had one lifetime sexual partner [6]. These factors point to an infectious aetiology, yet even in recent studies accounting for HPV infection, a role remains for the sexual activity, in particular before the age of 20, indicating some kind of a window of vulnerability. In the old days, marital status could be used as a proxy for sexual activity; this is no longer the case and detailed assessment of each patient's sexual activity is warranted [27].

Reproductive life is also linked to the risk of cervical cancer, with no influence of hormone-related determinants such as age at menarche or menopause, or characteristics of menses but, on the contrary, pregnancies do have an impact. Multiparity is a consistently-found risk factor, with women having had several full-term pregnancies carrying a higher risk. The role of multiple traumas to the cervix has been hypothesised. In one study, the age at last pregnancy was also found as a risk factor, at least for cancer occurring in women less than 45 years old [29].

The effect of oral contraceptive (OC) use on cervical cancer occurrence is particularly difficult to study. OC use is associated with characteristics of sexual life and screening behaviour which need to be controlled in the analysis [34]. Nevertheless, most of the available cohort or case-control studies are in favour of some increased risk, in particular when oral contraceptives are used for a long duration [22]. This is true for cervical dysplasia, carcinoma in situ and invasive cancer, and reinforces the credibility of the association, which has also been found in studies checking for HPV. In some studies, use of OC at an early age was linked to higher risk, even after adjustment for duration [12, 14]. In this issue the most important aspect is the link between histological type and OC. Risk seems to be clearer for adenocarcinoma than for squamous cell neoplasias [25, 41], although the results are not fully consistent [22]. Given the hormonodependance of adenocarcinoma, such an association makes sense and should be further explored, in particular since this histological type is on the increase.

Other hormonal products have also been evaluated, such as injectable contraceptives, where several studies found some increased risk - although not always statistically significant. In contrast, menopausal hormonal replacement therapy is not associated with risk [22].

Both descriptive and aetiologic studies have consistently found cervical cancer to be associated with deprivation, low social and educational status, as well as ethnicity and residence in low income countries [33, 34].

■ Human papilloma viruses

HPV now by far represents the strongest risk factor for cervical cancer and is even considered as a cause of the disease [21], some qualifying it as necessary [18].

More than 80 types of HPV are known, including at least 30 that are found in the genital tract. More than 20 animal papilloma viruses also exist. The usual classification is a function of the nucleotide sequences in five taxonomic groups, non phenotypically homogeneous. Two groups correspond to the majority of HPV. Over the years, methods of detection of viral DNA have become ever more sophisticated and, in parallel, the evaluation of the risk of cervical cancer as a function of HPV infection has improved.

HPV may be seen as a sexually-transmitted agent, although other modalities of infection also exist. In general, the primo-infection follows the onset of sexual activity and each sexual encounter augments the risk of infection. The acute manifestation of infection is the appearance of genital warts. It is estimated that about 1% of sexually active adults in the United States have clinical warts, whereas 15% or more have a subclinical infection. The highest rates of infection are found in young adults 18 to 28 years of age [24]. Most common genital HPV may also be found in non-genital sites, such as the mouth, fingers and skin in general, but also the lungs, in particular in newborns. Some data indicate an increasing trend of genital warts from the 50s to the 70s in the United States, corresponding to a period of more frequent sexually-transmitted diseases. Similar results have also been found in the United Kingdom. The role that increasing HPV infection may play in increasing rates of cervical cancer in young women is suggestive. This is further reinforced by the notion that viral HPV DNA is extremely frequent in low-grade cervical intra-epithelial neoplasia and quasi-constant in invasive tumours [21].

Many epidemiological studies are available and they are concordant. At the time the International Agency for Research on Cancer decided to evaluate the carcinogenic potential of HPV, more than 100 studies were already available. Almost all found a risk, and for the majority of studies, relative risks are extremely high. Yet, two periods can be clearly distinguished. The first corresponds to early studies having used non-PCR methods to detect HPV-16, or its nearest surrogate. The odds ratios (OR), used as estimates of relative risk (RR), are greater than 1, with the majority of values between 5 and 100. More recent studies, carried out with PCR methods, yield estimates between 5 and 500 [21]. Values of this magnitude are exceedingly rare in epidemiological studies, with the exception of viral agents. They strongly support the role of HPV as a cause of invasive cervical cancer. Other arguments in favour of this association come from the natural history of the disease and from molecular epidemiology. The infection by HPV precedes the occurrence of the tumour. The risk factors for HPV infection are similar to those for cervical cancer [26]. At the molecular level, the role of specific viral antigens differs between warts and cancers. HPV has been described as having a promoting effect on cellular proliferation, as well as being an inductor of chromosomal instability, and being capable of permitting cellular immortalisation in vitro. In addition, two oncoproteins, E6 and E7, interfere with the normal functions of negative cellular regulators, p53 and pRB [39].

Some co-factors may intervene, including hormones such as glucocorticoids or progesterone, and other viruses, such as Herpes Simplex Virus (HSV) [12] and Human Immunodeficiency Virus (HIV) [37]. Other sexually-transmitted agents, such as Neisseria gonorrhoeae and Chlamydia trachomatis, may also play a role [13].

In 1995, the conclusions of the IARC Monographs were already clear. The evidence was considered sufficient for the carcinogenicity in humans of HPV types 16 and 18. There was evidence suggesting the lack of carcinogenicity to the cervix in humans of HPV types 6 and 11, and there was limited evidence for the carcinogenicity in humans of some other HPV types. Although HPV cannot infect animals, some animal papilloma viruses cause cancer in their natural host. The overall evaluation was therefore that HPV types 16 and 18 are carcinogenic to humans (group 1), HPV types 31 and 33 are probably carcinogenic to humans (group 2A), and some HPV types other than 16, 18, 31 and 33 are possibly carcinogenic to humans (group 2B). The carcinogenicity of HPV types 16 and 18 is supported by experimental evidence that proteins of these viruses interfere with the functions of cellular regulatory pathways [21].

Since the publication of the Monograph, further studies have appeared, reinforcing the causal nature of the association between HPV and cervical cancer in many populations of the world, such as the Philippines [28], Thailand [9] and Morocco [8]. The most recent data also seems to implicate types other than 16 and 18 in cervical carcinogenesis.

■ Tobacco

Tobacco use has often been advanced as a possible risk factor for cervical cancer. The association was deemed weak and difficult to interpret due to confounding by sexual activity. Yet, several studies have demonstrated a link between smoking and high-grade cervical neoplasia [7, 20] as well as between smoking and condyloma acuminatum [16]. In a study of invasive cervical cancer, the association remained even after control for HPV infection. In fact, the risk linked to tobacco use was higher for HPV + than HPV- women [12]. Tobacco could act through its immuno-suppressive effect, leading to more active chronic infection and its accompanying inflammation.

Conclusion

Although its incidence and mortality are decreasing, cervical cancer remains an important cause of female morbidity and mortality. Cervical cancer has too long been considered as a social stigma for women of lower social class, as well as bearing the weight of its link with sexual activity. Today, we have a unique and challenging opportunity to develop a strategy aimed at preventing this still too frequent cancer, based on immunisation and the education of women.

References

[1] Beral V, Hermon C, Muñoz N, Devesa SS. Cervical cancer. *Cancer Surv* 1994 ; 19-20 : 265-285

[2] Berrino F, Capocaccia R, Estève J, Gatta G, Hakulinen T, Micheli A et al. Cervix uteri. In : Survival of cancer patients in Europe: the Eurocare-2 study. Lyon : International Agency for Research on Cancer, 1999 ; n° 151 : 314-323

[3] Berrino F, Sant M, Verdecchia A, Capocaccia R, Hakulinen T, Estève J. Cervix uteri. In : Survival of cancer patients in Europe: the Eurocare study. Lyon : International Agency for Research on Cancer, 1995 ; n° 132 : 266-278

[4] Blohmer JU, Schmalisch G, Klette I, Grineisen Y, Kohls A, Guski H et al. Increased incidence of cervical intraepithelial neoplasia in young women in the Mitte district, Berlin, Germany. *Acta Cytol* 1999 ; 43 : 195-200

[5] Bosch FX, Muñoz N, DeSanjosé S, Izarzugaza I, Gili M, Viladiu P et al. Risk factors for cervical cancer in Colombia and Spain. *Int J Cancer* 1992 ; 52 : 750-758

[6] Brinton LA, Reeves WC, Brenes MM, Herrero R, Gaitan E, Tenorio F et al. The male factor in the etiology of cervical cancer among sexually monogamous women. *Int J Cancer* 1989 ; 44 : 199-203

[7] Brisson J, Morin C, Fortier M, Roy M, Bouchard C, Leclerc J et al. Risk factors for cervical intraepithelial neoplasia: differences between low- and high-grade lesions. *Am J Epidemiol* 1994 ; 140 : 700-710

[8] Chaouki N, Bosch FX, Muñoz N, Meijer CJ, El Gueddari B, ElGhazi A et al. The viral origin of cervical cancer in Rabat, Morocco. *Int J Cancer* 1998 ; 75 : 546-554

[9] Chichareon S, Herrero R, Muñoz N, Bosch FX, Jacobs MV, Deacon J et al. Risk factors for cervical cancer in Thailand: a case-control study. *J Natl Cancer Inst* 1998 ; 90 : 50-57

[10] Ciatto S, Cecchini S, Iossa A, Grazzini G, Bonardi R, Zappa M et al. Trends in cervical cancer incidence in the district of Florence. *Eur J Cancer* 1995 ; 31A : 354-355

[11] Coleman MP, Estève J, Damiecki P, Arslan A, Renard H. Chapter 18: Cervix uteri. In : Trends in cancer incidence and mortality. Lyon : International Agency for Research on Cancer, 1993 ; n° 121 : 433-454

[12] Daling JR, Madeleine MM, McKnight B, Carter JJ, Wipf GC, Ashley R et al. The relationship of human papillomavirus-related cervical tumors to cigarette smoking, oral contraceptive use, and prior herpes simplex virus type 2 infection. *Cancer Epidemiol Biomarkers Prev* 1996 ; 5 : 541-548

[13] DeSanjosé S, Muñoz N, Bosch FX, Reimann K, Pedersen NS, Orfila J et al. Sexually transmitted agents and cervical neoplasia in Colombia and Spain. *Int J Cancer* 1994 ; 56 : 358-363

[14] Ebeling K, Nischan P, Schindler C. Use of oral contraceptives and risk of invasive cervical cancer in previously screened women. *Int J Cancer* 1987 ; 39 : 427-430

[15] Eide TJ. Cancer of the uterine cervix in Norway by histologic type, 1970-84. *J Natl Cancer Inst* 1987 ; 79 : 199-205

[16] Feldman JG, Chirgwin K, Dehovitz JA, Minkoff H. The association of smoking and risk of condyloma acuminatum in women. *Obstet Gynecol* 1997 ; 89 : 346-350

[17] Ferlay J, Black RJ, Pisani P, Valdivieso MT, Parkin DM. Eucan 90: Cancer in the European Union. Lyon : International Agency for Research on Cancer, 1996 ; n° 1 : 1-50

[18] Franco EL, Rohan TE, Villa LL. Epidemiologic evidence and human papillomavirus infection as a necessary cause of cervical cancer. *J Natl Cancer Inst* 1999 ; 91 : 506-511

[19] Gibson L, Spiegelhalter DJ, Camilleri-Ferrante C, Day NE. Trends in invasive cervical cancer incidence in East Anglia from 1971 to 1993. *J Med Screen* 1997 ; 4 : 44-48

[20] Gram IT, Austin H, Stalsberg H. Cigarette smoking and the incidence of cervical intraepithelial neoplasia, grade III, and cancer of the cervix uteri. *Am J Epidemiol* 1992 ; 135 : 341-346

[21] International Agency for Research on Cancer. IARC Monographs on the evaluation of carcinogenic risks to humans. Vol 64: Human papillomaviruses. Lyon : International Agency for Research on Cancer, 1995 ; 1-409

[22] International Agency for Research on Cancer. IARC Monographs on the evaluation of carcinogenic risks to humans. vol 72: Hormonal contraception and post-menopausal hormonal therapy. Lyon : International Agency for Research on Cancer, 1999 : 1-660

[23] Kjaer SK, Dahl C, Engholm G, Bock JE, Lynge E, Jensen OM. Case-control study of risk factors for cervical neoplasia in Denmark. II. Role of sexual activity, reproductive factors, and venereal infections. *Cancer Causes Control* 1992 ; 3 : 339-348

[24] Koutsky L. Epidemiology of genital human papillomavirus infection. *Am J Med* 1997 ; 102 (suppl 5A) : 3-8

[25] Lacey JV Jr, Brinton LA, Abbas FM, Barnes WA, Gravitt PE, Greenberg MD et al. Oral contraceptives as risk factors for cervical adenocarcinomas and squamous cell carcinomas. *Cancer Epidemiol Biomarkers Prev* 1999 : 8 : 1079-1085

[26] Muñoz N, Kato I, Bosch FX, Eluf-Neto J, De Sanjosé S, Ascunce N et al. Risk factors for HPV DNA detection in middle-aged women. *Sex Transm Dis* 1996 ; 23 : 504-510

[27] Murphy MF, Goldblatt PO, Mant D. Marital stability and cancer of the uterine cervix: changing patterns in post-war Britain. *Int J Epidemiol* 1993 ; 22 : 385-392

[28] Ngelangel C, Muñoz N, Bosch FX, Limson GM, Festin MR, Deacon J et al. Causes of cervical cancer in the Philippines: a case-control study. *J Natl Cancer Inst* 1998 ; 90 : 43-49

[29] Parazzini F, Chatenoud L, LaVecchia C, Negri E, Franceschi S, Bolis G. Determinants of risk of invasive cervical cancer in young women. *Br J Cancer* 1998 ; 77 : 838-841

[30] Parkin DM, Läärä E, Muir CS. Estimates of the worldwide frequency of sixteen major cancers in 1980. *Int J Cancer* 1988 ; 41 : 184-197

[31] Parkin DM, Pisani P, Ferlay J. Estimates of the worldwide incidence of eighteen major cancers in 1985. *Int J Cancer* 1993 ; 54 : 594-606

[32] Parkin DM, Pisani P, Ferlay J. Estimates of the worldwide incidence of 25 major cancers in 1990. *Int J Cancer* 1999 ; 80 : 827-841

[33] Parkin DM, Whelan SL, Ferlay J, Raymond L, Young J. Cervix uteri cancer. In : Cancer incidence in five continents. vol VII. Lyon : International Agency for Research on Cancer, 1997 ; n° 143 : 862-863, 1012-1013

[34] Schiffman MH, Brinton LA, Devesa SS, Fraumeni JF Jr. Cervical cancer. In : Schottenfeld D, Fraumeni JF Jr eds. Cancer: epidemiology and prevention. New York : Oxford University Press, 1996 : 1090-1116

[35] Skegg DC, Corwin PA, Paul C, Doll R. Importance of the male factor in cancer of the cervix. *Lancet* 1982 ; 2 : 581-583

[36] Sparen P, Gustafsson L, Friberg LG, Ponten J, Bergstrom R, Adami HO. Improved control of invasive cervical cancer in Sweden over six decades by earlier clinical detection and better treatment. *J Clin Oncol* 1995 ; 13 : 715-725

[37] Spitzer M. Lower genital tract intraepithelial neoplasia in HIV-infected women: guidelines for evaluation and management. *Obstet Gynecol Surv* 1999 ; 54 : 131-137

[38] Stockton D, Cooper P, Lonsdale RN. Changing incidence of invasive adenocarcinoma of the uterine cervix in East Anglia. *J Med Screen* 1997 ; 4 : 40-43

[39] Storey A, Thomas M, Kalita A, Harwood C, Gardiol D, Mantovani F et al. Role of a p53 polymorphism in the development of human papillomavirus-associated cancer. *Nature* 1998 ; 393 : 229-234

[40] Swerdlow AJ, Dos Santos Silva I, Reid A, Qiao Z, Brewster DH, Arrundale J. Trends in cancer incidence and mortality in Scotland: description and possible explanations. *Br J Cancer* 1998 ; 77 (suppl 3) : 1-54

[41] Ursin G, Peters RK, Henderson BE, D'Ablaing G 3rd, Monroe KR, Pike MC. Oral contraceptive use and adeno-carcinoma of cervix. *Lancet* 1994 ; 344 : 1390-1394

[42] World Health Organization. The world health report 1998. Life in the twenty-first century: a vision for all. Geneva : World Health Organization, 1998 : 1-230

[43] World Health Organization. The world health report 1999. Making a difference. Geneva : World Health Organization, 1999 : 1-131

Chapter 2

Problems in screening of cervical carcinoma

Anders Norström, Thomas Rådberg

A Norström, M.D., Ph.D.
T Rådberg, M.D., Ph.D.
Department of Obstetrics and Gynecology, Sahlgrenska University Hospital, S-413 45 Göteborg, Sweden.

Problems in screening of cervical carcinoma

A Norström, T Rådberg

Abstract. — *All systemised experiences of organised cervical cancer screening reveal a considerable reduction in both incidence and mortality of cervical carcinoma, although no randomised studies have proved their effectiveness. Epidemiological and experimental studies have established human papilloma virus (HPV) as the primary aetiological factor and the oncogenic subtypes have been identified. The present paper reviews the natural course of cervical precancerous lesions and HPV infections. Problems in cytological screening, such as terminology, population targeting, screening intervals, follow-up and treatment of cervical neoplasia are discussed. The importance of high coverage of the targeted population, optimal screening intervals and correct follow-up of atypical smears to avoid failures in a screening organisation is stressed. New techniques such as liquid-based cytology, thin layer preparations and automated devices are discussed as ways to reduce both the rate of false negative and false positive smears. Arguments are presented for the use of HPV testing in primary screening and in triage of equivocal smears to increase sensitivity and cost-effectiveness.*

Keywords: cancer prevention, cervical cancer screening, cervical intraepithelial neoplasia, cytology, human papilloma virus.

Introduction

World-wide efforts are steadily being made to reduce the cancer burden. The strategy in achieving this goal has several facets: to reduce the incidence of cancer by preventive measures, enabling early detection of the disease; to create effective therapy; and to offer proper palliative therapy and pain relief. The implementation of these measures depends on the attitudes of public health authorities as well as of the public and is directed by political, social, cultural and economic conditions. Cervical cancer fulfils established criteria for disease screening: it is a fairly common disease with serious consequences; its aetiology and natural history are known and it is possible to intervene effectively during its precancerous stages. In addition, screening can be performed with the use of a simple and reliable test: for decades, the Papanicolaou (Pap) test has contributed to a substantial reduction of the cancer burden in terms of reduced incidence and mortalilty of cervical cancer, as well as to a shift from advanced to early stages of the disease.

■ Effects of screening on cervical cancer incidence and mortality

It must be pointed out that in countries with long-established and well-organised screening, its value cannot be evaluated just in terms of reduced incidence of cervical cancer. An early indicator of the effectiveness of cervical screening is the change in cancer stage distribution due to a shift from advanced forms of this disease to early invasive stages [12]. Thus, an increasing number of women with early invasive cancers will be diagnosed. Many of them can be treated with simple conisation to preserve fertility, implying a screening success in terms of cost and quality of life.

In countries that have implemented organised screening programmes, a substantial reduction in both incidence and mortality of cervical cancer has been reported. In Sweden, after the introduction of organised screening at the beginning of the 60s, the incidence of cervical cancer was reduced by 60% and mortality by 40% [21]. Similar trends have been reported in other Nordic countries that introduced early nation-wide organised screening for cervical cancer. Iceland recently reported a 76% reduction in mortality and a 67% reduction of incidence in cervical cancer over the period 1986-1995 [31]. Similar effects of cervical screening were observed in Finland, whereas the reductions in incidence and mortality in cervical cancer were fewer in Denmark, which had a national screening coverage of only 45% in 1991, as well as in Norway, where organised screening was non-existent until 1994. In Norway (as compared to Sweden with an established screening programme), the incidence of cervical cancer was reduced at a considerably lower rate, in spite of the fact that the number of Pap smears per woman was similar, due to spontaneous (opportunistic) screening. This indicates that organised screening is more effective in reducing the risk of cervical cancer than spontaneous screening.

■ Cervical cancer aetiology

During recent years, epidemiological and experimental studies have established that the human papilloma virus (HPV) is the most important aetiological factor of pre-invasive and invasive cervical cancer. Sexually-transmitted HPV first infects the epithelial parabasal cells of the transformation zone (TZ). As soon as the HPV DNA is integrated into the host genome, oncoproteins encoded by the viral E6 and E7 genes are expressed and may inactivate the host suppressor proteins p53 and pRb respectively, thereby transforming an infected cell into a malignant phenotype. The mutations are permanent, extending viability of virally infected cells and allowing them to multiply in an uncontrolled way. It is likely that the expression of HPV genes is more prominent in rapidly dividing cells, which are more subject to chromosomal damage. Cell proliferation and cell repair induced by infection, trauma and hormonal factors could enhance this process and explain how other epidemiological risk factors, such as other sexually-transmitted diseases or many pregnancies at a young age, may contribute to the development of neoplastic disease. The HPV infection is associated with typical changes, which are first recognised in the cytoplasm and later, on integration of the viral genome, with nuclear changes and atypia, detected in the PAP smear as koilocytes.

More than 80 types of HPV have been identified by polymerase-chain reaction (PCR) based detection methods, and more than 30 of these have been isolated in the genital epithelium. Although HPV is unequivocally the main factor in cervical carcinogenesis, the oncogenic potential varies between different subtypes. HPV 16, 18, 45 and 56 are high-risk viruses, producing oncoproteins and found in high-grade cervical intraepithelial neoplasia (CIN) and most cancers. HPV 31, 33, 35, 39, 51, 52, 58, 61 represent an intermediate risk (high-grade CIN and some cancers), whereas HPV 6, 11, 30, 42-44 are considered to be low-risk viruses (genital warts and low-grade CIN). HPV has been detected in up to 95% of cervical cancer tumours, among which HPV 16 is preferentially isolated in squamous cells and HPV 18 in adeno- or adenosquamous cancers. The fact that HPV is not detected in all cervical cancer tumours may be due to mutations induced by HPV viruses not as yet characterised, or to other non HPV-related mutations of the host cell genome [5].

It has been suggested that HPV 18 related lesions are more aggressive and progress to invasive cancer directly from low-grade lesions. The adenocancers are often poorly differentiated and may be diagnosed more often in young women who have even had a normal Pap smear in the three years preceding diagnosis. Whether these observations do reflect a fast-progressing cancer disease per se or that adenocarcinomas usually start in endocervical glands high in the cervical canal and do not shed a sufficient number of cells to be detected in a Pap smear is still an open question.

As will be discussed, low-risk as well as high-risk HPV related precancerous lesions may regress spontaneously. Thus, it is obvious that other factors are interacting in malignant transformation. Hormonal factors, e.g. high parity or long-term use of oral contraceptives, have emerged as cofactors in HPV positive women. It has been suggested that constituents of cigarette smoke (e.g. cotinine, nicotine) may exert mitogenic, carcinogenic effects and/or impair local immune defense. The importance of the local immune system is further underlined by the higher risk of HPV infection, CIN and progression of CIN in immuno-compromised women and the association between cervical neoplasia and impaired, cell mediated immunity [5, 27, 34].

■ Pre-invasive cervical lesions: nomenclature

The function and reliability of a cervical screening programme is highly dependent on an accurate diagnostic language based on strict adherence to diagnostic criteria. Uniform terminology, locally, regionally and nationally, improves communication at all levels of the screening programme, reduces the risks of misinterpretation, and facilitates a proper, data-based registration of observations, follow-up and treatment as well as comparisons between different laboratories.

In 1973, the CIN classification was developed to replace the former descriptive classification of mild, moderate, severe dysplasia and carcinoma in situ (CIS) [29], and it

Table I. Natural history of cervical intraepithelial neoplasia (CIN) and human papillomavirus (HPV) lesions. Table compiled from Östör [26] and Syrjänen [33].

	Regress	Persistence	Progress to CIN III	Invasion
HPV-NCIN	80 %	15 %	5 %	0 %
CIN I	57 %	32 %	11 %	1 %
CIN II	43 %	35 %	22 %	5 %
CIN III	32 %	56 %		> 12 %

HPV-NCIN : HPV lesion without concomitant CIN.

is in use in many countries today. CIN I and CIN II correspond to the previously-named mild and moderate dysplasia, whereas CIN III covers the previous severe dysplasia and CIS. The CIN classification was originally intended for histology, but is nowadays commonly used for cytology, enabling an easier comparison of Pap smears and biopsy specimens. In 1988 the Bethesda System of classification was presented [23]. According to this system, squamous cell lesions (SIL) are separated into low-grade squamous cell lesions including koilocytosis (LSIL, corresponding to CIN I with the addition of koilocytosis) and high-grade squamous cell lesions (HSIL, corresponding to CIN II and III). ASCUS, according to the Bethesda classification, means atypical squamous cells of uncertain significance. ASCUS will identify women having a greater than background risk for concurrent and under-diagnosed SIL. Glandular epithelial lesions are separated into AGUS (glandular cells of uncertain significance) and AIS (adenocarcinoma in situ). AGUS applies to glandular cells that "demonstrate changes beyond those typical of benign reactive processes, yet that are insufficient for a diagnosis of adenocarcinoma." In the Bethesda system, there is no diagnosis for glandular dysplasia. Therefore, it is not surprising that up to 20% of precancerous and even cancerous lesions are detected on follow-up of women with AGUS [17]. According to the Bethesda system, the cytopathological report should include a statement on the adequacy of the specimens for diagnostic evaluation. Even though the Bethesda system may fail in defining the microscopical criteria of an adequate smear, it points out to smear takers and clinicians the importance of adequacy which should be registered and reported as a measure of quality assurance.

■ Cervical cancer: natural history

The guidelines for follow-up after detection of an atypical smear or treatment of a CIN are based on epidemiological data and knowledge of the natural course of pre-invasive lesions. Many studies attempting to describe the natural history of cervical cancer precursors have been published since the 50s. Östör's excellent review of these reports found a spontaneous regression rate of 57% for CIN I and a progression rate to CIN III and invasive cancer of 11% and 1%, respectively [26]. Generally, similar figures have been reported in studies estimating risks of progression of CIN I/CIN II lesions associated with HPV, although high-risk HPV per se increases the progression rate *(table I)*. It has also been reported that the regression rate increases with the extent of the follow-up time, whereas lesions tending to progress, appear to advance rapidly during the first 2 years of follow-up [7, 26].

The maximum incidence and prevalence of CIS occur at 30-34 years of age, though a significant number of CIS cases do appear among women in their 60s. The cumulative incidence of CIS is far higher than the cumulative incidence of invasive cervical cancer, indicating that even CIS might have a potential for spontaneous regression *(table I)*. CIS can be detected for several years before it progresses to invasive cancer, with an estimated latent period of 10 years [13].

Knowledge of the natural behaviour of premalignant cervical lesions certainly serves as a guide in the setting up of a screening programme and intervention, but is, however, insufficient in predicting the outcome of the disease in the individual woman.

Fundamentals of a cervical cancer screening programme

A screening programme is equally dependent on every single link in the chain: from invitation of the targeted population, cell sampling, laboratory results and reports, to follow-up and treatment. Causes of failure can be summarised in order of importance: 1) failure to reach the women at risk; 2) inadequate follow-up of abnormal smears; 3) long screening intervals; 4) false negative smear results (sampling as well as laboratory errors) [8]. Unfortunately, women with epidemiological high-risk factors have been known to be more prone to neglect invitations to screening. Therefore, the only factors that can easily be used as a basis for inviting women to an organised screening programme are age and screening history, enabling the identification of drop-outs and their re-invitation. As a screening organisation develops, coverage increases and, consequently, inadequate or insufficient follow-up and false-negative smear results become relatively more important.

■ Target population age groups

Very few cancers are seen in Western Europe before the age of 25-30 years and low-grade lesions, which are likely to regress spontaneously, are common below the age of 25. It has therefore been inferred that screening should start after the age of 25. However, in many regions, including all the Nordic countries except Finland, the incidence of invasive cancer - although low - is increasing in the 20-29 age group. Furthermore, in follow-up studies from Iceland, the proportion of women needing colposcopy and histological evaluation was as high in the 20-24 as in the 25-29 age groups. These observations imply that screening should start between 20 to 25 years. The Swedish Board of Health and Welfare recommends starting at the age of 23. It has been suggested that screening could stop at the age of 50, provided at least three negative smears have been obtained earlier. Up to the age of 70-75, incidence and mortality decrease in a population that has been screened at younger ages. However, the protective effect against invasive disease that is exerted by a short time span between negative smears is stronger than merely the numbers of negative smears taken earlier. Theoretical calculations of register data and life expectancies at different ages in England and Wales have also implied that increasing the upper screening age to 65-69 would save more life years than focusing on younger ages, and would prevent half of the present deaths from cervical cancer up to the age of 80 and beyond [19]. However, there are such marked differences in the age spectrum, even in close geographical and ethnic populations such as in the Nordic countries, so that each programme must be designed, carefully monitored and adjusted to local trends [30]. As a result of increased migration, many women are lost to primary screening as well as follow-up after an equivocal smear. Therefore, before the decision is taken to stop screening women between 60-69, there should be efforts made to identify and reach women who have never been screened or who have had previous questionable smears [3, 4].

Table II. Reduction in the cumulative incidence of cervical cancer according to the proportion of the population covered by screening in relation to the interval between smear tests. From Miller AB [22], p 53.

Frequency of smear tests	Proportion of population screened (%)	Reduction of cumulative incidence (%)
1 year	20	19
2 years	30	28
3 years	40	37
5 years	50	42
10 years	80	51

■ Screening intervals

It has been suggested that intervals between smears should not exceed five years and not be shorter than 2-3 years. The national screening programmes in the different Nordic countries with intervals between 3 and 5 years appear to be equally protective. However, in Finland, which uses a 5 year interval programme, there are widespread and uncontrolled spontaneous screenings and therefore, it is not possible to assess if 5 year intervals are really equally effective. The International Agency for Research on Cancer (IARC) Collaborative Study calculated that screening at 3 year intervals between the ages of 20-64 and 25–64 would be equally effective, both resulting in a > 90% incidence reduction. On the other hand, starting at 30 with a 3 year interval or using 5 year intervals between 20-64 would yield only a < 85% reduction. In this context it must be stressed that it is far more important to reach a high proportion of the targeted population and screen them less frequently than to reach a smaller proportion for frequent screening *(table II)*. Thus, "high coverage/low intensity" is more cost-effective than "low coverage/high intensity" (the latter being the situation in countries where spontaneous or opportunistic screening dominates without sufficient integration in a less organised screening programme, such as the case in Norway before 1994. On the other hand, in Iceland and to some extent in Norway, the screening organisation is enhanced by fortunate conditions such as a small, stationary and homogenous population. Here, screening is conducted in close collaboration with the central statistical register, allowing complete integration of organised and spontaneous smear taking; there is only one cytopathological laboratory using a uniform terminology; the population is informed about screening through leaflets, newspapers and other media; GPs and other health professionals are regularly informed about attendance rates, non-attending women, quality of samples, abnormalities, follow-up and treatment. These strategies have lead to a coverage of 83% of the targeted population, a follow-up compliance of abnormal smears of 98% which has resulted in reductions of 76% in mortality and incidence of 67% in cervical cancer over the 10 year period 1986-1995 [32].

■ Cell sampling

The reported rate of false negative smears varies greatly in studies, partly depending on the different operative definitions used. For instance, the proportion of women with invasive disease in spite of a recent negative smear is obviously overestimated compared to the rate calculated from the actual presence of CIN or cancer based on biopsies taken at the same time as the negative smear. Regardless of definition, the rate of false negative smears has been calculated to be in the range of < 10-40% [14].

The major cause appears to be errors in sampling and/or preparation procedures which account for 50-75% of all false negatives [15]. In this context, it must be stressed that the size and the histological type as well as the location of the lesion have an important influence on the rate of false negative smears. As mentioned above, early endocervical cancers, adeno– or adenosqamous cancers shed fewer cells or cells that are more easily overlooked. The combined use of a classic Ayres spatula and endocervical brushes reduces the proportion of smears lacking endocervical cells, resulting in smears which are supposedly more representative of the transformation zone. This procedure has also been reported to increase the number of dyskaryotic smears in screening samples. However, it is well recognised that only a small and selected proportion of sampled cells are actually transposed to the glass slide. Furthermore, suboptimal procedures of fixation impair conditions for accurate microscopic assessment of the sample. New technology, such as liquid-based cytology and/or thin-layer preparations, are thought to overcome some of these pitfalls and make the screening less dependent on the performance of the smear takers.

Using thin-layer technology, the sample is transferred into a transport preservative fluid (avoiding the negative influence of air-drying) to the laboratory. The presence of obscuring material, e.g. blood, mucus, cell debris, etc., can be removed, providing samples of "pure" and representative cells, which are more easily read by the cytotechnologist [15].

In a prospective multicentre study enrolling more than 7,000 women, there was an average 65% improvement using the thin-layer technique in detecting precancerous lesions as compared to conventional Pap smears. The techniques were equivalent in detecting benign cellular changes. The increased sensitivity of the thin layer preparation did not cause a loss in overall specificity. An additional advantage of the thin-layer slides is their usefulness in concomitant HPV testing [20].

Thus, thin-layer preparations yield superior sensitivity and higher specificity as compared to conventional slides. The drawbacks, however, are higher initial costs for training, as well as costs for sampling, transport and preparation.

■ Laboratory errors

The rate of smears misclassified by the laboratory can be defined in two ways: 1) a narrow definition, including missed low- and high-grade neoplastic lesions that are recognised on rescreening; 2) a broad definition, including ASCUS and AGUS smears and in certain studies also unsatisfactory smears.

Depending on the definition used, laboratory errors of between 5% to 20% have been reported [16, 18]. The main quality control measures for cytological laboratories include: 1) rescreening of all smears taken from women who developed invasive cancers. The results of this rescreening should be regularly compiled, analysed and reported to all personnel involved; 2) diagnostic tests and qualifying examinations for all personnel engaged in cytological diagnostics; 3) internal quality controls, which should include correlative analyses and distribution of cytological and histopathological diagnoses, including even ASCUS/AGUS, koilocytic and unsatisfactory smears. Reports should be specified and made available to users; 4) new technologies which have been suggested as helpful means for internal control such as HPV testing in reviewing the accuracy of koilocytotic changes. Automated screening devices have been used in attempts to increase both the sensitivity and specificity of cytology. Automated cervical cytology has been utilised in up front primary screening, in rescreening to identify false negative smears, and as a quality control modality after manual screening. Meta-analyses of five investigations applying the PAPNET system indicated that this technique, compared to manual screening, identifies 20% more abnormalities, has two times fewer false negatives and reclassifies as abnormal one third of manually screened negative slides [1]. The new screening, technologies appear to increase the sensitivity of cervical screening effectively, but costs are still a significant hinderance to their more widespread use. On the other hand, it has been calculated that screening with any of the new techniques, the thin- layer preparation included, every 3 years, was lower in cost per year of life saved than screening with conventional Pap smears every 2 years [6]. Automated techniques may help increase the capacity of a laboratory, enabling the cytotechnologist to focus on questionable samples and are certainly a means for quality control. Although used in the rescreening and quality control of manually screened smears, automated scanning devices have to be intermittently controlled by the cytotechnologists, who therefore retain their role as the gold standard in cervical screening.

■ Follow-up

Adequate follow-up is of paramount significance in any screening programme. With an increasing number of smears with minor and borderline atypia, less costly follow-up procedures have been called for. These include surveillance by "cytology-only" in primary health care and "see-and-treat" office procedures; the former method risking delayed diagnoses of early invasive disease, the latter risking over-treatment of non-neoplastic lesions. The experience of many countries is reassuring, at least in young women, as ASCUS and LSIL smears can be managed by cytological surveillance over two years [11, 31]. If all the smears are normal, these women can be safely brought back to standard screening programmes. If, however, a second atypical smear is obtained, immediate colposcopic and histopathological evaluation should be performed. A population of highly-compliant women is a prerequisite for this approach, and/or an organisation that can immediately identify and recall drop-outs. In women aged over 25-30 years with earlier atypical smears, as in all women with HSIL (or CIN II-III), immediate colposcopy and biopsy as well as subsequent or simultaneous treatment ("see-and-treat" excision) are mandatory. For the triage of smears showing ASCUS/AGUS or minor atypias, the use of HPV technology has been advocated. Using semi-quantitative HPV testing with probes against single or combined high risk HPV types, about 60% or more of the cases with CIN II-III can be identified, reaching a sensitivity of over 90% if combined with a second smear. As is the case with the above-mentioned new technologies in cytology, triage by HPV testing will add more costs to the follow-up until long-term results are convincing enough to abandon the established cytological surveillance.

■ Post-treatment follow-up

In a well-screened population, there is an increasing number of women with new cancers who have been previously evaluated because of atypical smears. Even after classical high conisations, there is an increased risk of invasive cervical cancer for as long as 20 years after treatment [28]. Hence, follow-up after treatment is an important part of all screening programmes. After an initial period of two years, cytological surveillance at 2-3 year intervals for at least two decades to reveal residual disease is meaningful and will reduce mortality and treatment costs for these women. However, it may not be equally effective in reducing the incidence of invasive cancers. This view is strongly supported by a recent observation in a Swedish county with intensive screening which showed this category of women to have half of all the new cervical cancers, which were almost all found in early, preclinical stages, as opposed to the other half, which were usually diagnosed in late stage I-III [2]. The role of other methods than cytology, such as colposcopy and HPV testing, in treatment follow-up is not yet established. Both methods appear to increase the detection rate of residual CIN soon after treatment [10]. However, whether they are cost-effective in long-term follow-up is not yet known.

Screening for HPV in conjunction with Pap smear screening

In the light of today's knowledge that high-risk HPV can be detected in nearly 100% of women with CIS or cancer, and that there is a hundred-fold greater risk of high-risk HPV positive women with normal Pap smears developing CIN, the inclusion of HPV testing in a cervical screening programme appears to be a rational decision. HPV testing may be helpful in detecting high-risk cases among women having ASCUS and even among women with normal smears. Several methods are currently in use to recognise the target (viral) nucleic acid sequences through complementary nucleic acid sequences (probes). The PCR technique enables the identification of very low levels of viral nucleic acids. The Hybrid Capture method is sensitive, accurately quantitative and suitable for screening, being available in standardised kit format.

HPV infections are common among young women and, in most cases, will resolve spontaneously, as will CIN in young women (up to 80%). In women > 35 years of age, however, the regression rate of premalignant lesions is only 40% [33]. Both retrospective and prospective studies indicate that women with abnormal cytology but no or low-risk HPV infection do not show progression to CIN III, whereas the existence of high-risk HPV appears to be a dominant factor in progression to HSIL (CIN II-III) [25]. There are strong indications that combining a Pap smear with HPV testing could increase the effectiveness of a screening programme: HPV negative women with normal smears could be screened less frequently with preserved security, whereas high-risk, HPV positive women with negative smears would be subjected to rescreening at a higher intensity. Women with CIN I or ASCUS and no or low-risk HPV would not necessarily have to be referred for treatment, but followed conservatively, whereas those with high-risk HPV should be referred for further colposcopy and biopsy. HPV screening in conjunction with PAP smears can separate women into low and high risk groups and could advocate screening at longer intervals. Detection of high-risk HPV in women having mild to moderate dyskaryosis also predicts progression to CIN III better than a second Pap smear. Thus, the additional costs for the HPV testing could thereby be compensated for economically [25]. HPV tests are reproducible and objective, eliminating human error and the subjectivity associated with the interpretation of Pap smears. HPV testing needs a limited number of qualified technicians and has therefore been suggested as an alternative screening instrument. HPV technology is evolving and further data on specificity and sensitivity of novel methods are probably still to come. Cost-benefit aspects must be considered before introducing routine HPV testing in a population with well-organised Pap smear screening programmes.

Endocervical precancerous lesions

Conventional cell sampling has inherent shortcomings in the detection of atypical endocervical cells: the cells may not be shed sufficiently to be detected in a smear and atypical cells may be located, uni- or multifocally, deep in the cervical glands, thereby escaping the cytobrush. There is not yet concensus as to whether or not there is a progression from mild cellular atypia to a cancer in situ lesion (CIN III or AIS) via a stage of moderate atypia. Some authors claim that different grades of endocervical intraepithelial neoplasia can be detected with the same accuracy as that of detecting squamous lesions. According to other investigators, CIN/AIS develops abruptly from benign glandular epithelium without a transition through glandular dysplasia. A fast transition might explain higher rates of false negatives of glandular atypias and their being missed more frequently than squamous cell lesions at screening at 3 year intervals. HPV 18 is the predominant HPV subtype in pre-invasive and invasive glandular lesions. An early integration of the HPV 18 genome in the host cell genome may underly a rapid transition from benign to neoplastic cells. Hormonal factors, such as the use of oral contraceptives (OC), are considered to be related to the development of cervical adenocarcinoma. In this context, progestogens competing for the glucocorticoid receptor in HPV DNA may impair the viral regulatory gene. The glandular cells infected by HPV do not undergo similar morphololological changes of koilocytotic atypia as HPV infected, squamous cells do. On the other hand, glandular lesions are co-existent with squamous cell lesions in more than 50% of cases and might be detected while treating a superficial disease.

Psychological aspects of screening

The extent to which women participate in screening is associated with age, education, marital status and other socio-economic factors. Non-compliers are usually older, single, poor and have a higher incidence and mortality risk. Adequate information given in leaflets and media about the aim and the positive effects of cervical cancer screening, not only in detecting cancer but also, and particularly, in preventing its development, will certainly encourage attendance. At least 5% of the women participating in cervical screening will be confronted with the report of an abnormal smear. Their fear and anxiety must be dealt with in an understanding and sympathetic way to ensure compliance in follow-up, and professionally to avoid over-consumption of health resources [24].

Concluding remarks

By using Pap smear screening in an organised protocol, both the incidence and mortality of squamous cell carcinomas can be effectively reduced. Earlier as well as recent experiences in Canada and Western Europe support the views published in the Europe Against Cancer Programme [9]. A screening programme should be continuously monitored, using a comprehensive person based register enabling a coverage of > 85% of women aged 25-65 within intervals of < 5 years. Provided at least 5 normal smears have been obtained from a given screening, intensity can be reduced to intervals of 5 years after the age of 50, and stop at 60-65. Efforts to reach women above the age of 55-60 who have never participated in screening or failed to follow-up after an abnormal smear are probably more rewarding in the near future than introducing new technology. The proposed application of HPV testing to select which women should be screened more intensely and those who can safely be screened less intensely, e.g at 5 year intervals before the age of 40, still needs to be confirmed in on-going trials before it can be generally recommended. However, in the follow-up of women with low-grade or equivocal smears, the combined use of HPV testing will increase effectiveness compared to cytological surveillance alone.

References

[1] Abulafia O, Sherer DM. Automated cervical cytology: meta-analyses of the performance of the PAPNET system. *Obst Gynecol Surevey* 1999 ; 4 : 253-264

[2] Andersson-Ellström A, Seidal T, Grannas M, Hagmar B. The Pap-smear history of women with invasive sqamous carcinoma. A case-control study from Sweden. *Acta Obstet Gynecol Scand* 2000 ; 79 : 221-226

[3] Andrae B, Smith P. Clinical impact of quality assurance in an organized cervical screening program. *Acta Obstet Gynecol Scand* 1999 ; 78 : 429-435

[4] Benedet JL, Miller DM, Nickerson KG. Results of conservative management of cervical intraepithelial neoplasia. *Obstet Gynecol* 1992 ; 79 : 105-110

[5] Bornstein J, Rahat MA, Abramovici H. Etiology of cervical cancer: current concepts. *Obstet Gynecol Survey* 1995 ; 50 : 146-154

[6] Brown AD, Garber AM. Cost-effectiveness of 3 methods to enhance the sensitivity of Papanicolaou testing. *J Am Med Assoc* 1999 ; 281 : 347-353

[7] Campion MJ, McCance DJ, Cuzick J, Singer A. Progressive potential of mild cervical atypia: prospective cytological, colposcopic and virological study. *Lancet* 1986 ; 2 : 237-240

[8] Chamberlain J. Reasons that some screening programmes fail to control cervical cancer. In : Hakama M, Miller AB, Day NE ed. Screening for cervical cancer of the uterine cervix. *IARC Sci Publ* 1986 ; 76 : 161-168

[9] Coleman D, Day N, Douglas G, Farmery E, Lynge E, Philip J et al. European guidelines for quality assurance in cervical cancer screening. Europe against cancer programme. *Eur J Cancer* 1993 ; 29 (suppl A) : S1-S38

[10] Elfgren K, Bistoletti P, Dillner L, Walboomers JM, Meijer CJ, Dillner J. Conization for cervical intraepithelial neoplasia is followed by disappearance of human papillomavirus deoxyribonucleic acid and a decline in serum and cervical mucus antibodies against human papillomavirus antigens. *Am J Obstet Gynecol* 1996 ; 174 : 937-942

[11] Ferenczy A, Jenson AB. Tissue effects and host response. The key to the rational triage of cervical neoplasia. *Obstet Gynecol Clin North Am* 1996 ; 23 : 759-782

[12] Gibson L, Spiegelhalter DJ, Camilleri-Ferrante C, Day NE. Trends in invasive cervical cancer incidence in East Anglia from 1971 to 1993. *J Med Screen* 1997 ; 4 : 44-48

[13] Gustafsson L, Pontén J, Bergström R, Adami HO. International incidence rates of invasive cervical cancer before cytological screening. *Int J Cancer* 1997 ; 71 : 159-165

[14] Hakama M, Miller AB, Day NE. Screening for Cancer of the Uterine Cervix. Lyon : International Agency for Research on Cancer, 1986

[15] Hutchinson ML, Isenstein LM, Goodman A, Hurley AA, Douglas KL, Mui KK et al. Homogeneous sampling account for the increased diagnostic accuracy using the ThinPrep processor. *Am J Clin Pathol* 1994 ; 101 : 215-219

[16] Jones BA. Rescreening in gynecologic cytology. Rescreening of 3762 previous cases for current high-grade squamous intraepithelial lesions and carcinoma- a College of American Pathologists Q-Probes study of 312 institutions. *Arch Pathol Lab Med* 1995 ; 119 : 1097-1103

[17] Kennedy AW, Salmieri SS, Wirth SL, Biscotti CV, Tuason LJ, Travarca MJ et al. Results of the clinical evaluation of atypical glandular cells of undetermined significance (AGCUS) detected on cervical cytology screening. *Gynecol Oncol* 1996 ; 63 : 14-18

[18] Koss LG. Cervical (Pap) smear. New directions. *Cancer* 1993 ; 71 : 1406-1412

[19] Law MR, Morris JK, Wald NJ. The importance of age in screening for cancer. *J Med Screen* 1999 ; 6 : 16-20

[20] Linder J. Liquid-based cytology: comparison of ThinPrep 2000 with conventionally prepared Pap smears. In : Franco E, Monsenego J ed. New Developments in CervicalCancer Screening and Prevention. (Franco et Monsenego) 1998 : 284-293

[21] Mälck CG, Jonsson H, Lenner P. Pap smear screening and changes in cervical cancer mortality in Sweden. *Int J Epidemiol* 1985 ; 14 : 521-527

[22] Miller AB. Cervical Cancer Screening Programmes. Managerial Guidelines. World Health Organization, Geneva. 1992

[23] National Cancer Institute Workshop. The 1988 Bethesda System for reporting cervical/vaginal cytological diagnoses. *JAMA* 1989 ; 262 : 931-934

[24] Nicoll PM, Narayan KV, Paterson JG. Cervical screening cancer: women's knowledge, attitudes and preferences. *Health Bull (Edinburgh)* 1991 ; 49 : 184-190

[25] Nobbenhuis MA, Walboomers JMM, Helmerhorst TJ, Rozendaal L, Remmink AJ, Risse EK et al. Relation of human papillomavirus status to cervical lesions and consequences for cervical-cancer screening: a prospective study. *Lancet* 1999 ; 354 : 20-25

[26] Östör AG. Natural history of cervical intraepithelial neoplasia: a critical review. *Int J Gynecol Pathol* 1993 ; 12 : 186-192

[27] Petry KU, Scheffel D, Bode U, Gabrysiak T, Kochel H, Jupsch E et al. Cellular immunodeficiency enhances the progression of human papilloma-associated cervical lesions. *Int J Cancer* 1994 ; 57 : 836-40

[28] Pettersson F, Silverswärd C. Diagnosis and management of cervical abnormalities. *IARC Sci Publ* 1986 ; 76 : 221-237

[29] Richart RM. Cervical intraepithelial neoplasia. *Pathol Assoc* 1973 ; 8 : 301-328

[30] Sasieni P, Cuzick J, Farmery E. Accelerated decline in cervical cancer mortality in England and Wales. *Lancet* 1995 ; 346 : 1566-1567

[31] Sigurdsson K. The Icelandic and Nordic cervical screening programs: trends in incidence and mortality rates through 1995. *Acta Obstet Gynecol Scand* 1999 ; 78 : 478-485

[32] Sigurdsson K. Trends in cervical intra-epithelial neoplasia in Iceland through 1995: evaluation of targeted age groups and screening intervals. *Acta Obstet Gynecol Scand* 1999 ; 78 : 486-492

[33] Syrjänen KJ. Spontaneous evolution of intraepithelial lesions according to the grade and type of implicated human papillomavirus (HPV). *Eur J Obstetr Reprod Biol* 1996 ; 65 : 45-53

[34] Van Oortmarssen GJ, Habbema JD. Epidemiological evidence for age-dependent regression of pre-invasive cervical cancer. *Br J Cancer* 1991 ; 64 : 559-565

Chapter 3

Problems in the diagnosis of invasive cervical carcinoma

Mahmood I Shafi, Joseph A Jordan

MI Shafi, MD DA MRCOG, Consultant Gynaecological Surgeon and Oncologist.
JA , Jordan, MD FRCOG, Consultant Gynaecologist and Medical Director.
Birmingham Women's Hospital, Edgbaston, Birmingham B15 2TG, United Kingdom.

Problems in the diagnosis of invasive cervical carcinoma

MI Shafi, JA Jordan

Abstract. — The appropriate and timely investigation of women with possible cervical cancer is important. Colposcopy will detect early invasive lesions but ultimately the diagnosis is histological. The type of biopsy used for diagnosis should be carefully considered to provide maximal information and the possibility of affecting a cure in very early lesions. Generally, where doubt exists, local excisional treatments are safer than ablative procedures. The pathological interpretation of the biopsy is of paramount importance and forms the basis of further management. In some cases of early invasive disease, a carefully performed excisional biopsy may be the only treatment required.

Keywords: colposcopy, biopsy, diagnosis.

Introduction

Cervical cancer is common – particularly in underdeveloped countries. Presentation differs markedly in developed and underdeveloped countries – in the former, the majority of cases (75%) present at an early stage where cure may be expected with treatment. In contrast, presentation in underdeveloped countries is usually late and often equates to mortality since a cure cannot be anticipated. The major determinant of the presentation difference is the educational level of the women and their empowerment. In developed countries, women either present early with their symptoms or take part in cervical cytology screening programmes. Such screening programmes are not often feasible in the majority of underdeveloped countries, where health demands differ.

Cervical cancers often present with symptoms which warrant further investigation. In others, the presentation is due to abnormal cervical cytology and the diagnosis suspected at the time of colposcopic examination of the cervix. Whatever the presentation, diagnosis is dependent upon taking an appropriate biopsy that will confirm, and in some situations treat, the condition [3].

The staging of cervical cancer is clinical, but in the early stages, the interpretation of the pathological specimen is paramount. This is why, when cervical cancer is suspected, the woman should be seen by those experienced in investigation, since information obtained at an early management phase will impact on further treatments.

Factors indicating need for further investigation

Cervical cytology is not diagnostic and is merely a screening technique for pre-invasive cervical disease. It can suggest an invasive process if highly atypical cells are present in the smear associated with tumour debris. The chance of finding invasive disease in an asymptomatic woman presenting with abnormal cervical cytology is dependent on the degree of cytological abnormality. Careful colposcopic assessment needs to be undertaken to identify those women with early invasive lesions. Even if the cervical smear is negative, there is a chance that invasive disease may be present, especially if the lesion is necrotic and does not desquamate cells. Therefore, if the appearance of the cervix is abnormal, or the texture/consistency raises the possibility of malignancy, referral for further investigation should be made, irrespective of the cervical smear result.

Cervical cytological features that would suggest the possibility of early invasive disease are:

- Tendency to form large sheets of cells rather than strings.
- Smaller, paler staining nuclei/cells.
- Cytoplasmic differentiation.
- Projections to cytoplasm, sometimes keratinised.
- Increased pleomorphism.
- More obvious nuclear abnormalities.
- Loss of round appearance to cells.

In those women presenting with symptoms, the most common symptoms are:

– Postcoital bleeding.

– Postmenopausal bleeding.

– Offensive vaginal discharge.

The discharge associated with cervical cancer is due to tumour necrosis. It is often yellowish in nature, thin, sometimes bloodstained or foul smelling. Symptoms associated with cervical cancer occur earlier in lesions on the ectocervix as compared to lesions confined to the endocervical canal. With more advanced lesions, bleeding and discharge can be significant and unpredictable.

Women with advanced cervical malignancy may have other associated symptoms due to disease extension into other structures and the general affects of advanced neoplasia. These symptoms include backache, leg pain/oedema, haematuria, bowel changes, malaise and weight loss. The pain associated with advanced cervical cancer is due to involvement of the lumbosacral plexus. Leg oedema is secondary to lymphatic involvement or vascular obstruction. When there is extension to the bladder and rectum, there may be symptoms of frequency, dysuria, haematuria, diarrhoea, tenesmus or rectal bleeding. If fistula formation results, then there will be incontinence of either urine or faeces. Malaise is associated with anaemia and impaired renal function.

If vaginal bleeding occurs during pregnancy, while the most common reason will be pregnancy-related, it must be remembered that malignant cervical lesions can and do occur and therefore should be systematically excluded.

Colposcopic features associated with malignancy

Some lesions will obviously be apparent at the time of colposcopic examination, displaying either an exophytic or an ulcerative lesion. Others may be much harder to identify and require skilled colposcopic assessment. Extended (classical) colposcopy is particularly useful [1]. Excess cervical mucus can be gently removed and the cervix cleaned with a saline-soaked wool swab. Following this, acetic acid and Schiller's iodine test may be used. The latter two stains make assessment of the angio-architecture difficult if the saline technique has been omitted.

Using saline solution, atypical cervical vessels can be visualised, particularly if a green filter is used at high magnification [4]. The red capillaries and vessels appear darker and stand out more clearly. Atypical vessels are focally sited within the cervix and differ from the mosaic, punctation or delicately branching vessels seen with cervical intra-epithelial neoplasia. With invasive disease, the vessels appear irregular with abruptly changing courses. Several characteristic forms are described as "comma", "corkscrew" and "spaghetti-like" forms. These atypical vessels are of uneven calibre and generally coarser than normal vessels. These vessels may appear and disappear abruptly as part of their course in neoplastic disease.

Early invasive lesions do not always have atypical vessel patterns recognised colposcopically. Features that are associated with a higher likelihood of malignant change are large lesions with coarse changes of aceto-whiteness, mosaicism and punctation. Other features to note are an irregular surface, and lesions extending into the cervical canal, making full colposcopic assessment impossible.

Even in those where disease is easily visualised, colposcopy is useful in delineating the extent of the disease, particularly in terms of vaginal extension. This can influence further treatment by accurately recording the extent of invasive and pre-invasive disease.

Approach to diagnosis

Tissue from the suspected area of the cervix is required to make a histological diagnosis of malignancy. Neither cytology nor colposcopy can make the diagnosis, but they can indicate the appropriate investigation and the size of the biopsy required.

The types of biopsy used in diagnosis are:

– Colposcopically-directed punch biopsies.

– Excisional biopsies.

– Diathermy loop excision, large loop excision of transformation zone (LLETZ), loop electrodiathermy excision procedure (LEEP).

– Laser excision.

– Knife cone biopsy.

– Wedge biopsy.

– Hysterectomy.

Whichever biopsy is used, it should be deep enough to establish the diagnosis of invasion, and an endocervical canal curettage is useful if an endocervical canal lesion is suspected. In some countries, endocervical curettage is not usually performed, and if endocervical malignancy is suspected, then the cervical canal is biopsied using one of the above methods. If invasive disease is suspected, then a colposcopically-directed punch biopsy may well be inadequate to confirm the nature of the disease. The larger biopsy techniques have the advantage of being able to remove the transformation zone in its entirety, making histological interpretation much more accurate and definitive [2, 7]. If early invasive disease is suspected, a knife cone biopsy has the advantage that the excision margins are less likely to be distorted with heat/diathermy artefact and, therefore, histological interpretation is improved. A wedge biopsy is useful when trying to confirm or exclude invasion and is generally undertaken under general anaesthesia. The major indication for this procedure would be the assessment of the pregnant woman with suspected cervical malignancy. This is because the associated morbidity is less than that for a conisation and the diagnostic accuracy is superior to a colposcopically-directed biopsy.

The "suspicious" cervix

Lesions on the cervix may present as an exophytic, cauliflower-like lesion. This is often associated with necrosis and contact bleeding. These tumours grow either in a polypoid or papillary fashion and can attain considerable bulk but only infiltrate the cervical stroma to a limited degree. These exophytic lesions tend to show less tendency to involvement of the parametria. Other tumours may burrow under the surface, creating an ulcerated lesion. If the tumour arises in the endocervical canal, then a firm, hard, barrel-shaped tumour results. Neither the site of origin nor the pattern of growth of cervical tumours offers any guidance as to their histological nature.

Where there is local extension of the tumour, it can spread laterally, inferiorly or superiorly. With lateral spread, the paracervical lymphatics and parametria are involved. If this process is extensive, then disease can extend to the pelvic side-walls. This type of spread can involve the distal ureters, causing obstruction and renal impairment. With inferior extension, the vaginal epithelium and stroma can be involved. With extensive vaginal involvement of the subvaginal lymphatics, there can be spread into the lower third of the vagina and occasionally metastatic spread to the inguinal lymphatics. Cervical cancer may also extend superiorly to involve the proximal endocervix and the lower uterine segment. These tumours are often large in nature, and magnetic resonance imaging is ideal for further investigations.

When there is lymphatic spread, this is primarily to the internal iliac, obturator, external iliac and common iliac lymph nodes. Cervical cancer can spread from the pelvis to involve the para-aortic lymph nodes and eventually the supraclavicular nodes.

Cervical stump carcinoma

This is unlikely to develop in a woman who has had subtotal hysterectomy with an adequate cervical screening history. Presentation is similar to that in patients with the uterus intact. If suspected, an adequate biopsy is taken before definitive treatment can be undertaken.

Unsuspected carcinoma in hysterectomy specimen

If a woman is having a simple hysterectomy for benign conditions, then an adequate cervical screening history should exist. If recent cervical cytology has been abnormal, then a pre-operative colposcopic assessment is mandatory. Despite this, unsuspected cervical carcinoma may be found occasionally in women undergoing simple hysterectomy for a presumed benign disorder. Further treatment is based on detailed histological assessment of the surgical specimen and also patient factors. Many of these women will require adjuvant radiotherapy, although re-operation can be considered in selected cases [6].

Cervical cancer in pregnancy

Between 1-3% of all cervical cancers are diagnosed during pregnancy. The possibility of such a neoplasm is often overlooked in women presenting with vaginal bleeding in pregnancy, especially if this is recurrent, due to the assumption that bleeding is pregnancy-associated. Visualisation of the cervix and colposcopic assessment, if indicated, are important. If suspected, then an adequate diagnostic biopsy is warranted, accepting the higher risk of haemorrhage associated with such procedures. The timing of diagnosis can have significant implications for the pregnancy, and the mother needs to be fully involved in the decision-making process. There does not appear to be any worse prognosis with cervical cancers in pregnancy, but good data on the effects of delay in management are not available [8].

During pregnancy, any colposcopic examination will be complicated, as normal features are distorted due to pregnancy effects on the cervix [5]. Active squamous metaplasia, especially of the immature type, can present diagnostic difficulties. There is also excessive mucus production, poor access and patient discomfort as the pregnancy advances. The vascularity of the cervix is accentuated and the colposcopic impression is usually of a worse lesion than actually exists. This is why, in these situations, it is important for an experienced colposcopist to be available so that adequate assessment is undertaken without recourse to unnecessary intervention. Gentleness during the procedure is important, as well as adequate explanation to the woman, who will be anxious about the situation. If the sidewalls of the vagina are a problem in gaining access to the cervix, then a bivalve speculum with a surrounding condom or a finger from a rubber glove can be used. Any kind of biopsy is associated with increased risk of haemorrhage and should only be undertaken if malignancy is suspected. If bleeding does occur, then either simple pressure or sutures may be used to gain haemostasis.

Diagnostic difficulties

Two particular situations that cause diagnosis problems for colposcopists are: the "inflammatory" cervix, and the "wart-like" lesion. In those women with an inflamed-looking cervix, appropriate microbiological investigation is undertaken. If there is any doubt about the diagnosis, early recourse to biopsy of the cervix should be undertaken so as not to miss the invasive cervical lesion masquerading as an inflamed cervix.

Condylomata on the cervix are exophytic and the majority are easily diagnosed. A smear history is important prior to management. Occasionally, the surface of the condyloma may have "encephaloid" features with a whorled surface. In others, the surface may be hyperkeratotic, and in these circumstances histological diagnosis is essential. The differential diagnosis can include verrucous cervical carcinomas. Excisional methods of treatment are considered safer than ablative methods in these situations.

References

[1] Anderson M, Jordan J, Morse A, Sharp F. A text and atlas of integrated colposcopy. London : Chapman and Hall, 1992

[2] Bigrigg A, Haffenden DK, Sheehan AL, Codling BW, Read MD. Efficacy and safety of large-loop excision of the transformation zone. *Lancet* 1994 ; 343 : 32-34

[3] Kehoe S, Shafi MI. Update on cervical cancer. In : Studd JW ed. RCOG Yearbook. London : RCOG Publications, 1996

[4] Kraatz H. Farbfiltervorshaltung zur leichteren Erlernung der Kolposkopie. *Zentralbl Gynakol* 1939 ; 63 : 2307-2309

[5] Luesley DM. Difficult situations and management problems. In : Luesley DM, Shafi MI, Jordan JA eds. Handbook of colposcopy. London : Chapman and Hall, 1996

[6] Orr JW, Ball GC, Soong SJ. Surgical treatment of women found to have invasive cervical cancer at the time of total hysterectomy. *Obstet Gynecol* 1986 ; 68 : 353-356

[7] Prendiville W, Davies R,, Berry PJ. A low voltage diathermy loop for taking cervical biopsies: a qualitative comparison with punch biopsy forceps. *Br J Obstet Gynaecol* 1986 ; 93 : 773-776

[8] Sivanesaratnam V, Jayalakshmi P, Loo C. Surgical management of early invasive cervical cancer of the cervix associated with pregnancy. *Gynecol Oncol* 1993 ; 48 : 68-75

Chapter 4

Pathology of cervical carcinoma

Franck Fétissof

F Fétissof, Professor, Centre Hospitalier Universitaire, Hôpital Bretonneau, 2 bd Tonnellé, 37044 Tours Cedex 1, France.

Pathology of cervical carcinoma

F Fétissof

Abstract. — *The role of the pathologist in a multidisciplinary gynaecological oncology team is essential not only for establishing the diagnosis, but also for determining the prognostic factors that govern treatment. The WHO classification (1994) distinguishes squamous cell carcinomas which are the most common, adenocarcinomas which are increasing in incidence in young women, and other epithelial tumours. Secondary tumours in the cervix are rare. For each tumour, prognosis depends on the grade and on the FIGO clinical stage.*

Keywords: squamous cell carcinomas, adenocarcinomas, classifications, pathology.

General remarks: the role of the pathologist

Invasive carcinomas represent only some of the cervical tumours. They are infiltrating (primary or secondary) malignant epithelial tumours; only these will be discussed in this section. In particular, dysplasia (cervical intra-epithelial neoplasia (CIN), carcinoma in situ), adenocarcinomas in situ and malignant mesodermal mixed tumours will not be considered.

The clinical pathologist belongs to a multidisciplinary team in which he occupies a privileged position between the specimen taker, in this case the surgeon, and the therapist. He provides essential information for treatment and for diagnosis and prognostic features which are mainly based on the stage and on the grade associated with the histological appearance of the tumour.

■ The report

In his report, the pathologist must provide a diagnosis and two sets of prognostic information from which the tumour's stage and its histological grade can be established. At present, a major effort is being undertaken to standardise the reports. It is recommended that World Health Organisation (WHO) terminology be used. There are also a number of recommendations or protocols at local (oncology network), national and international levels concerning the management of specimens and the compilation of reports.

Each report must include the following information:

– macroscopic size of the tumour;
– histological type;
– grade (optional if squamous cell carcinoma);
– tumour spread;
– depth of tumour infiltration;
– width of tumour infiltration;
– extracervical spread (vagina, body of uterus, parametrium, etc.);
– vascular invasion;
– quality of resection borders (particularly the lower limit of resection);
– presence of lymph nodes and number of metastatic lymph nodes.

■ WHO classification

This is the reference classification. The latest edition (second edition) of the WHO classification of tumours of the female genital tract dates back to 1994. This classification combines tumours of the body of the uterus, gestational trophoblastic disease, tumours of the uterine cervix, vagina and vulva *(fig 1)*.

The tumours can be found in group 1, corresponding to primary tumours, and in group 5, corresponding to secondary tumours or metastases. In group 1, there are three subgroups corresponding to squamous lesions (1.1), glandular lesions (1.2), and other epithelial tumours (1.3). Each of these subgroups include squamous cell carcinomas

Tumour of the cervix

Primary epithelial (1)
tumour

Secondary epithelial tumour (5)

Other epithelial tumours. Varieties (1.3)(1-7)

Squamous lesion
(1.1)

Glandular lesion (1.2)

Squamous cell carcinoma (1.1.7)

Adenocarcinoma (1.2.6)

Variants 1.1.7 (1-6)

Variants 1.2.6 (1-5)

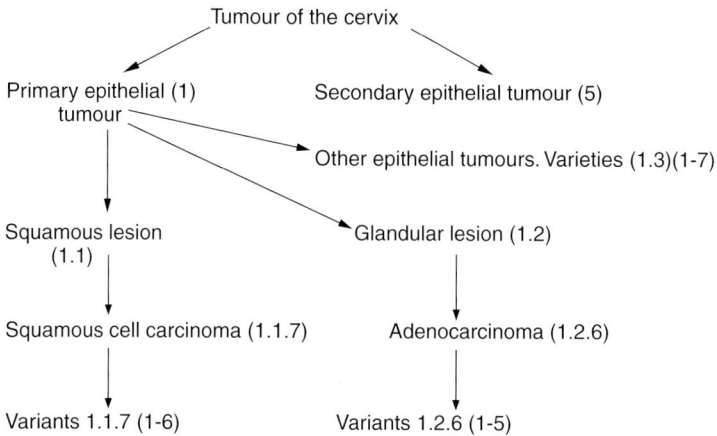

Figure 1. *Principle of the WHO classification of invasive carcinomas.*

Table I. Different types of squamous cell carcinomas.

Keratinising
Non-keratinising
Verrucous
Warty (condylomatous)
Papillary
Lympho-epithelioma-like carcinoma

Table II. Different types of adenocarcinomas.

Mucinous adenocarcinoma
Endocervical type
Intestinal type
Endometrioid adenocarcinoma
Clear cell adenocarcinoma
Serous adenocarcinoma
Mesonephric adenocarcinoma

(1.1.7) and variants (1.1.7 1-6), adenocarcinomas (1.2.6) and variants (1.2.6 1-5), and the different varieties of other epithelial tumours (1.3.1-7) *(tables I, II, III)*.

Identification of the tumour entities should not be based solely on morphological criteria, but should also be of prognostic or therapeutic value.

■ Grading

In general, grading is based on the morphological appearance of the tumour. Grading takes into account the differentiation of the tumour, its mitotic activity and cytological atypia.

Table III. Other epithelial tumours.

Adenosquamous carcinoma
Glassy cell carcinoma
Adenoid cystic carcinoma
Adenoid basal carcinoma
Carcinoid tumour
Small cell carcinoma
Undifferentiated carcinoma

Squamous cell carcinomas: there is no grading which is clearly correlated to prognosis. Grading is optional.

– Grade 1: well differentiated squamous carcinoma.
– Grade 2: moderately differentiated squamous carcinoma.
– Grade 3: poorly differentiated squamous carcinoma.
– Grade 4: undifferentiated carcinoma.

Adenocarcinomas: grading is of prognostic value; it takes the architecture of the tumour (glandular or papillary formations versus solid architecture) and cytological atypia into account.

– Grade 1: Minimal solid architecture < 10% solid area. Minor to moderate cytological atypia.
– Grade 2: Intermediate between grade 1 and grade 3: 10% to 50% solid area.
– Grade 3: Predominantly solid architecture > 50% solid area. Major cytological atypia.

Nuclear grading:

– non-atypical nucleus;
– very atypical nucleus (increased size, volume, condensed chromatin, prominent nucleolus);
– intermediate appearance.

■ TNM classification of malignant tumours

The latest Tumour, Nodule, Metastasis (TNM) and International Federation of Gynaecology and Obstetrics (FIGO) classifications (5th edition 1997) are summarised in table IV. They are the reference classifications for tumour staging. In his report, the pathologist must provide the information from which the stage can be established. This also involves prognostic factors related to the tumour stage (pTNM stage).

The information likely to be involved in this classification includes the depth of the infiltration (3 mm, 5 mm), the horizontal spread (7 mm), the size of the tumour (4 cm), its spread outside the body of the uterus (parametrium, vagina, pelvic wall, bladder, rectum). The histological examination of a pelvic lymphadenectomy must usually include at least 10 lymph nodes.

Micro-invasive squamous cell carcinoma [5, 19]

■ Concept of micro-invasive carcinoma

This is based on the possibility of identifying an infiltrating carcinomatous formation with an almost non-existent metastatic potential and with no effect on survival. Under

Table IV. Classification of malignant tumours - cervix uteri.

Cervix Uteri

(CIM-0 C53)

The definitions of T categories correspond to the nomenclature adopted by FIGO. Both classification systems are presented together for comparison.

Classification Rules

The classification only applies to carcinoma. Every case must be confirmed by histological evidence.

The required conditions for determination of T, N and M are as follows:

T Categories	clinical examination, cystoscopy* and imagery including urography
N Categories	clinical examination and imagery including urography and lymphangiography
M Categories	clinical examination and imagery

Note. *Cystoscopy is not necessary for a Tis.

Anatomic Localisation

1. Endocervix (C53.0)

2. Exocervix (C53.1)

Regional Adenopathies

Lymphatic invasion can concern the following nodes: paracervical, parametrial, external iliac, hypogastric (obturator), primitive iliac, presacral and latero-sacral.

TNM Clinical Classification

T - Primitive Tumour

TNM Categories			FIGO Stages		
TX					Insufficient information to categorise the primitive tumour
T0					No sign of primitive tumour
Tis			0		Carcinoma in situ
T1			1		The carcinoma is strictly confined to the cervix (extension to the corpus should be disregarded)
	T1a			IA	Micro-invasive carcinoma diagnosed only by histology. All macroscopically visible lesions – even with superficial invasion – are allocated to Stage T1b or IB
		T1a1		IA1	Measured stromal invasion ≤ 3 mm in depth and ≤ 7 mm in horizontal extension
		T1a2		IA2	Measured stromal invasion > 3 mm and ≤ 5 mm in depth and ≤ 7 mm in horizontal extension
					Note. The depth of invasion must not be greater than 5 mm from the base of the epithelium of the original tissue. Depth of invasion is defined as the measurement of the tumour from the epithelio-stromal junction of adjacent epithelial papillary stratum to the deepest invasion point. The invasion of vascular space – venous or lymphatic – does not modify the classification.
	T1b			IB	Clinically visible lesion limited to the cervix uteri or microscopic lesion $> $ T1a2
		T1b1		IB1	Clinically visible lesion ≤ 4 cm in its greatest diameter
		T1b2		IB2	Clinically visible lesion > 4 cm in its greatest diameter

Table IV. (con't.) Classification of malignant tumours - cervix uteri.

T2		II	Cervical carcinoma extending beyond the uterus but not to the pelvic wall or to the lower third of the vagina
	T2a	IIA	No parametrial invasion
	T2b	IIB	With parametrial invasion
T3		III	Cervical carcinoma extending to the pelvic wall and/or the lower third of the vagina, and/or with hydronephrosis or non-functioning kidney
	T3a	IIIA	Extending to the lower third of the vagina, but not to the pelvic wall
	T3b	IIIB	Extending to the pelvic wall and/or with hydronephrosis or non-functioning kidney
T4		IVA	Tumour extending to the *mucous membrane* of the bladder or rectum and/or extending beyond the true pelvis
			Note. The presence of a bullous oedema is not sufficient to categorise a tumour as T4.
			Note. The presence of an oily oedema is not sufficient to categorise a tumour as T4.
M1		IVB	Metastases spread to distant organs

N - Regional Adenopathies

NX	Insufficient information to categorise invasion of regional lymphatic nodes
N0	No sign of nodal invasion
N1	Signs of nodal invasion

M - Metastases to Distant Organs

MX	Insufficient information to categorise distant metastases
M0	No distant metastases
M1	Distant metastases

pTNM Histopathologic Classification

pT, pN and pM categories correspond to T, N and M categories.

pN0	The histological examination of a pelvic lymphadenectomy should normally include at least 10 lymphatic nodes.

these conditions, the therapeutic approach to this variety of infiltrating tumour would be similar to that of high grade intra-epithelial lesions (CIN3-carcinoma in situ) and would differ radically from that of other infiltrating carcinomas. This is the major benefit of distinguishing this group of micro-invasive carcinomas.

Metastatic potential is probably correlated to tumour volume. In practice, this is difficult to evaluate and can be more readily understood by the depth of the infiltration and the size of the tumour *(table V)*. The impact of the vascular invasion may also be considered. Conversely, the architecture of the lesion might not have a prognostic influence.

The prognostic value of vascular invasion is disputed: its presence may increase metastatic risk. However, vascular invasion increases with the depth of infiltration and under these conditions, it can be questioned as to whether or not it is a risk factor which is independent of the depth of infiltration. The prognostic value of vascular invasion appears greater for lesions measuring less than 3 mm in depth. The metastatic risk increases from 0-1% to 3.5%.

Table IV. (con't.) Classification of malignant tumours - cervix uteri.

Grouping by Stages			
Stage 0	Tis	N0	M0
Stage IA	T1a	N0	M0
Stage IA1	T1a1	N0	M0
Stage IA2	T1a2	N0	M0
Stage IB	T1b	N0	M0
Stage IB1	T1b1	N0	M0
Stage IB2	T1b2	N0	M0
Stage IIA	T2a	N0	M0
Stage IIB	T2b	N1	M0
Stage IIIA	T3a	N0	M0
Stage IIIB	T1	N1	M0
	T2	N1	M0
	T3a	N1	M0
	T3b	any N	M0
Stage IVA	T4	any N	M0
Stage IVB	any T	any N	M1

Summary				
TNM		**Cervix uteri**	**FIGO**	
Tis		In situ	0	
T1		Limited to uterus	1	
	T1a	Histological diagnosis only		IA
	T1a1	Depth = ≤ 3 mm, extension = ≤ 7 mm		IA1
	T1a2	Depth > 3-5 mm, extension ≤ 7 mm		IA2
	T1b	Clinically visible lesions > T1a2		IB
	T1b1	≤ 4 cm		IB1
	T1b2	> 4 cm		IB2
T2		Beyond uterus but not to pelvic wall or lower third of vagina	II	
	T2a	Parametrium intact	IIA	
	T2b	Parametrium invaded	IIB	
T3		Lower third of vagina/pelvic wall/hydronephrosis	III	
	T3a	Lower third of vagina	IIIA	
	T3b	Pelvic wall/hydronephrosis	IIIB	
T4		Mucous membrane of bladder/rectum beyond true pelvis	IVA	
M1		Distant metastases	IVB	

Table V. Correlation between the depth of infiltration, the presence of nodal metastases and vascular invasion.

Depth of infiltration	Nodal metastasis
< 1 mm	0.4%
3 mm	0-0.5%-0.9%
3.1-5 mm	5.3%-13.19%
< 5 mm	1%
Depth of infiltration	Vascular invasion
< 1 mm	0 to 8%
1 to 3 mm	9 to 29%
Stage IA2	39%

Table VI. Diagnostic stages.

Cytology → high-grade intra-epithelial lesion

↓

Colposcopy, biopsy → CIN2, CIN3

↓

Conisation   Complete examination of the specimen
                                              → Micro-invasive
                                                carcinoma
Hysterectomy   Lesion totally excised

■ Definition

A micro-invasive lesion can be defined as one in which neoplastic epithelium invades the stroma in one or more places to a depth of 3 mm or less, below the basement membrane of the epithelium; no lymphatic or blood vascular involvement is detected.

This diagnosis can only be made on the basis of a totally resected lesion, including its intra-epithelial component; it can therefore only be made after a complete histological examination of a conisation or a hysterectomy specimen *(table VI)*.

Micro-invasive carcinoma does not belong to a specific TNM category or FIGO stage. Micro-invasive carcinomas belong to the T1A category, and more specifically T1A1. There is however no absolute equivalence between T1A1 and micro-invasive carcinoma. In fact T1A1 tumours may exhibit vascular invasion and their width must not exceed 7 mm. Defined in this way, the micro-invasive carcinoma has no risk of metastasis or relapse and has no effect on survival.

■ Frequency and clinical features

The mean age of onset is 40 years (from 20 to 70 years). Eight to ten percent of invasive carcinomas are micro-invasive. They are present in 4% to 7% of conisation specimens for CIN. The incidence of micro-invasive carcinoma is 4.8/100,000 whereas that of CIN is 316/100,000.

Micro-invasive carcinoma is an asymptomatic lesion: the cervix has a normal appearance or exhibits only minor changes. Colposcopic examination reveals CIN features, but with a vascular network which is somewhat abnormal in places. Tumour infiltration of more than 1 mm is necessary to induce colposcopic changes suggestive of an invasive process.

Cytological examination cannot detect micro-invasion.

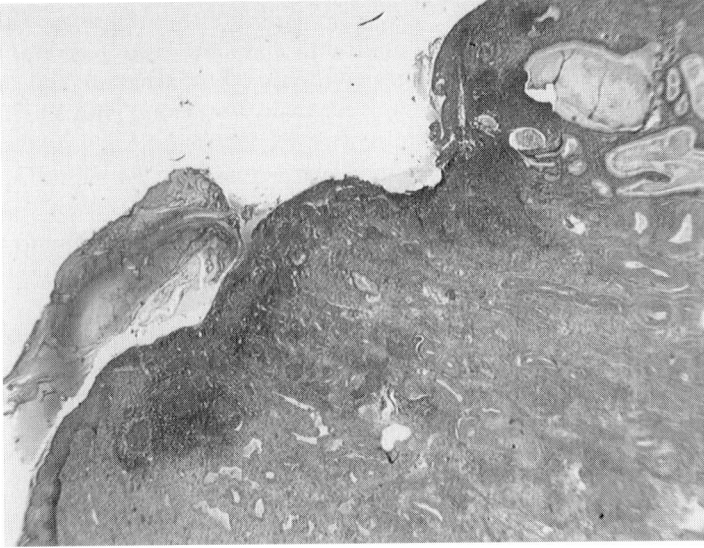

Figure 2. *Micro-invasive carcinoma. Carcinomatous infiltration is no more than 3 mm in depth with no vascular invasion.*

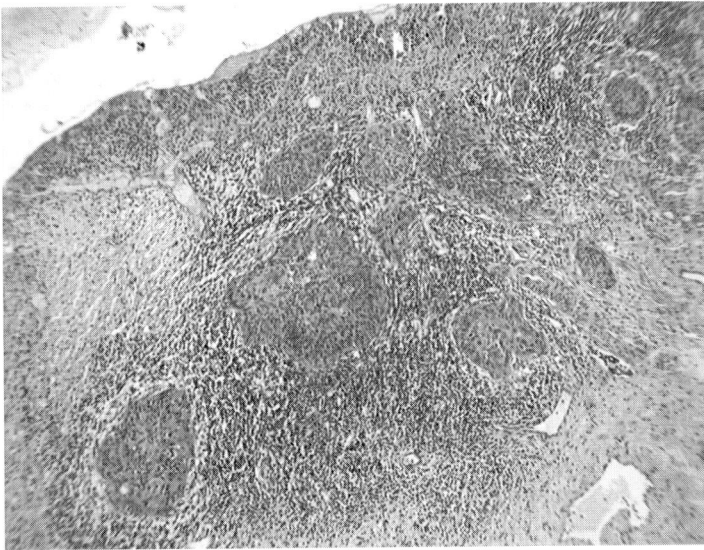

Figure 3. *Micro-invasive carcinoma (grossly magnified). This carcinoma develops from surface CIN. Note the inflammatory changes next to the invasive carcinomatous formations.*

■ Histological examination *(fig 2, 3)*

Histologically, the micro-invasive foci have irregular, jagged contours and the junction between the epithelium and connective tissue is blurred. The micro-invasive foci are often clearly differentiated and more mature than the rest of the lesion. The cells possess abundant eosinophilic cytoplasm with incipient signs of keratinisation. The nuclei are nucleolated. These major changes are indicative of infiltration. Other changes may be observed. Infiltration is associated with a desmoplastic reaction, rich in acid mucosubstances and with an inflammatory infiltrate. The epithelium appears scalloped and pleated. The micro-invasive carcinoma occurs in association with a high-grade CIN (low-grade, exceptionally).

The depth of infiltration is measured from its starting point in the surface epithelium or a gland.

Vascular invasion must be looked for, possibly using immunohistochemical techniques (Factor VIII, CD34, lectins, etc.).

Visualisation of the basement membrane by histochemical (reticulin) or immunohistochemical techniques (laminin, collagen IV, fibronectin) is of little value in that the basement membrane may be focally absent in a simple inflammatory process, and present when in contact with a highly differentiated invasive carcinoma [24].

The clinical pathology report must mention:

– the depth of the infiltration;

– the degree of lateral spread (in the form of a micro-invasive lesion or CIN);

– the quality of the resection;

– the investigation for vascular invasion.

■ Differential diagnosis

Micro-invasive carcinoma must be distinguished from:

– intraglandular spread of CIN or immature metaplasia;

– incarceration in the lamina propria of epithelial formations which were normal or dysplastic on a previous biopsy;

– CIN exhibiting fragmentation of the basement membrane, associated with an inflammatory process.

All these problems of differential diagnosis do not extend beyond the context of CIN and demonstrate the risk of over diagnosis of a micro-invasive carcinoma.

Micro-invasive carcinomas may benefit from conservative treatment (conisation or simple hysterectomy) as for CIN. For all other carcinomas that do not meet the strict definition of a micro-invasive carcinoma, particularly if there is vascular invasion, more radical treatment than that for usual invasive carcinomas must be considered.

Epidermoid or squamous cell carcinoma *(table VII)*

■ General remarks

Squamous cell carcinoma is the most common carcinoma of the genital region and particularly the uterine cervix. Its incidence is tending to diminish because of systematic cytological screening. However, there is a large disparity between rich and poor countries.

Conventionally, this tumour tends to be observed more frequently in elderly women. At present, an increased frequency has been observed in young women. Fifty percent of

Table VII. Types of squamous cell carcinoma.
1. Epithelial tumours and related lesions
1.1 Squamous lesions
1.1.7 Squamous cell carcinoma
1.1.7.1 Keratinising
1.1.7.2 Non-keratinising
1.1.7.3 Verrucous
1.1.7.4 Warty (condylomatous)
1.1.7.5 Papillary
1.1.7.6 Lympho-epithelioma-like carcinoma

cases are seen before the age of 50 and 25% before 35 years. The clinical expression depends on the size of the tumour and its stage. For advanced lesions, symptoms are abnormal vaginal bleeding (after intercourse), serosanguineous intermittent discharge or spotting, bloody malodorous discharge. Invasion of the bladder or rectum may be in the form of dysuria, haematuria or rectorrhagia. The earliest lesions may be totally asymptomatic and only detected at cytological screening [26]. The clinical phase may be separated from the subclinical phase by an interval of ten years or more.

Its frequency is correlated to the age of first intercourse, but also to multiparity, low economic level, many sexual partners and promiscuity of the male partner. Infiltrating squamous cell carcinoma is often associated with and preceded by CIN. It has the same epidemiological characteristics as CIN [6]. Fewer than 5% of CIN1 develop into squamous cell carcinoma; 2/3 of CIN3 develop into squamous cell carcinoma within 3 to 20 years. HPV is found in at least 80% of squamous cell carcinomas. Other viruses are sometimes mentioned (herpes virus II, EBV, HTLV-1, HIV) [23].

In a number of cases, squamous cell carcinoma develops without a precursor lesion, without associated CIN and without any association with HPV. Other aetiological factors have been implicated in the development of squamous cell carcinomas: smoking, oral contraception, diethylstilbestrol (DES), etc.

- Classic form

Macroscopic appearance

Incipient lesions may present in the form of a focal induration or an ulcerated or prominent lesion. In almost all cases, lesions develop over a transformation zone and spread, in varying degrees, over the rest of the exocervical surface. On colposcopic examination, infiltration may be suspected if there is an abnormal vascular network with tortuous and abnormally disposed vessels. As it develops, the lesion may present in an essentially infiltrating exophytic, polypoid or endophytic form. It should be noted that even a markedly developed lesion may be macroscopically almost undetectable.

Microscopic appearance

This carcinoma tends to resemble squamous epithelium and sometimes exhibits keratinisation. Conventionally a distinction is drawn between:

– a form with large keratinising cells;

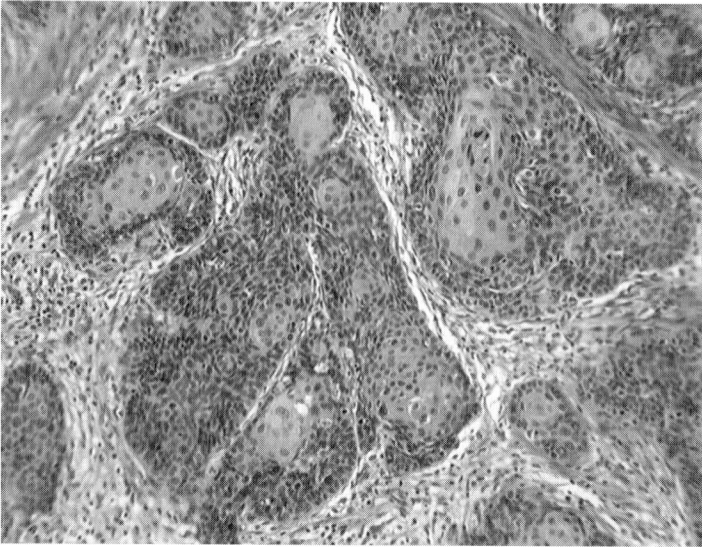

Figure 4. *Squamous cell carcinoma. A fairly differentiated carcinoma, with large, non-keratinising cells.*

– a form with large non-keratinising cells *(fig 4)*;

– a form with small cells.

Two forms are considered at present: keratinising and non-keratinising (the small cell form includes, at least in part, carcinomas with a neuro-endocrine differentiation). The appearance of these carcinomas also varies according to the degree of differentiation. Association with CIN is common. Some histological features may be reported: acantholysis with a "pseudoglandular pattern", amylosis deposits, infiltration by eosinophils. It is acceptable for an squamous cell carcinoma to include some cells with mucus droplets without suggesting a diagnosis of muco-epidermoid or adenosquamous carcinoma.

Ninety percent of cases are positive for carcino-embryonic antigen. Progesterone receptors may be present. Aneuploidy is the rule, but there is a high degree of heterogeneity within the same tumour (30% to 80% are aneuploid and 20% to 40% are diploid).

Outcome

Squamous cell carcinoma spreads directly into the adjacent tissues; firstly in the planes offering little resistance (perinervous, perivascular, pericervical, parametrium) and then attaining the ligaments, bone, etc. (It is disseminated lymphatically and more rarely haematogenically).

– Direct, local extension is to the vagina, corpus (endometrium and myometrium), parametrial soft tissue, lower urinary tract (ureter, bladder), rectum, uterosacral ligament, pelvic wall, bony pelvis.

– Lymphatic invasion occurs early and nodal metastases may be observed:

– 1st group affected: paracervical, hypogastric, obturator, iliac (internal, external, common).

– 2nd group affected: sacral, para-aortic, inguinal.

– More rarely: supradiaphragmatic, supraclavicular node.

– Nodal metastases are found in stage IB in 8% to 25% of cases, in stage II in 20% to 40% of cases and in stage III in 30% to 50% of cases.

– Visceral metastases are possible but rarer (despite the presence of vascular emboli in about 50% of cases), lung in 9% of cases and bone in 4% of cases.

– Ovarian metastases are rarer than with adenocarcinomas, but are nevertheless possible.

– Recurrences (essentially pelvic) occur within 2 years. Death may be related to peritonitis (obstruction and perforation of the colon), respiratory insufficiency (pulmonary metastases), cardiac insufficiency, thrombosis, embolism, haemorrhage, etc.

Prognosis [14, 21]

A number of prognostic factors of greater or lesser relevance have been advanced: stage, nodal metastases, tumour volume or size, depth of infiltration, vascular invasion, histological grade, type of squamous cell carcinoma, HPV status, flow cytometry, etc.

The stage is certainly the most important prognostic factor.

Five-year survival is 90% to 95% for stage I; 50% to 70% for stage II; 30% to 35% for stage III and 20% for stage IV.

Nodal metastases reduce survival, irrespective of the stage. However, the risk of nodal metastases is correlated to the stage. Five-year survival for stage I is 95% if there are no nodal metastases, 62% if there is one and 17% if there are two.

For a specific stage, the tumour volume, depth of infiltration and vascular invasion may have a prognostic influence.

There is no conclusive demonstration that a histological grading system reliably predicts prognosis. The keratinising forms appear more radio resistant than the non-keratinising forms. Five-year survival for stage I treated by radiotherapy is 54% for the keratinising form and 84% for the non-keratinising form. Grade 3 recurs more frequently and has a shorter survival time. Absence of HPV might be a poor prognostic factor.

The clinical importance of tumour ploidy is currently unclear. The prognosis is the same for aneuploid and diploid tumours.

▪ Verrucous carcinoma (giant condyloma acuminatum of Busckhe and Lowenstein)

Macroscopically this is a large, warty, bulbous lesion with a fungal appearance. The deep margin is sharply circumscribed. This sessile tumour is widely implanted in the cervix.

Microscopically, it consists of papillomatous or undulating hyperplastic squamous epithelium *(fig 5)*. The lesion bristles with papillary projections with or without keratinisation. The base of the tumour is composed of invasive nests of epithelium that are broad and expansile with a well-circumscribed pushing margin. At the deep margin, large bulbous masses invade along a wide front. The squamous epithelium is clearly differentiated without cytological atypia. It sometimes involves a deeply invasive lesion, even extending into the endometrium or adjacent pelvic tissues.

This tumour does not exhibit any metastatic spread. However locally, it may involve an extensively infiltrating, destructive tumour.

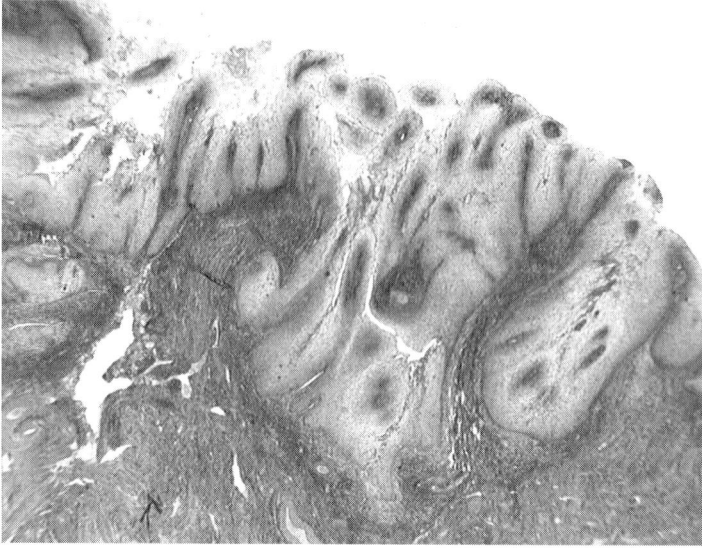

Figure 5. *Verrucous carcinoma. A well differentiated variant of squamous cell carcinoma. Note the papilloma-tous surface.*

This tumour is associated with HPV 6/11.

Its treatment is based on extensive resection which is not always possible. Irradiation may cause acceleration of growth and metastatic development.

At the outset, diagnosis from biopsies is difficult. It requires close clinical and pathological co-operation. It is often only possible on the hysterectomy specimen. Differential diagnosis concerns condyloma acuminatum particularly with large exophytic condylomata with glandular involvement, a highly differentiated squamous cell carcinoma and a warty (condylomatous) carcinoma. Finally, we should point out the possible association of verrucous and squamous cell carcinoma.

■ Warty (condylomatous) carcinoma

This variety of squamous cell carcinoma has a striking condylomatous or warty appearance. It presents as a classically appearing condyloma extending deeply into the endocervical canal, associated in some cases with invasive cancer. This tumour form seems to be less aggressive than the classic squamous cell carcinoma.

The differential diagnosis essentially includes verrucous carcinoma.

■ Papillary carcinoma [28]

This variant of invasive squamous cell carcinoma has a superficial resemblance to transitional cell carcinoma. This tumour is composed superficially of papillary vegetations. These are lined with epithelium exhibiting the appearance of a high-grade intra-epithelial lesion; focal squamous differentiation may be observed. Carcinomatous infiltration can be found at the base of the lesion or along the axis of the papillae; for this reason, a papillary lesion containing marked atypia should be considered invasive until proven otherwise.

Table VIII. Types and frequence of adenocarcinoma.
1 Epithelial tumours and related lesions
1.2 Glandular lesions
1.2.6 Adenocarcinoma
1.2.6.1 Mucinous adenocarcinoma 50 to 60%
1.2.6.1.1 Endocervical type
1.2.6.1.2 Intestinal type
1.2.6.2 Endometroid adenocarcinoma 30%
1.2.6.3 Clear cell adenocarcinoma 5 to 10%
1.2.6.4 Serous adenocarcinoma < 5%
1.2.6.5 Mesonephric adenocarcinoma < 5%

If there is no infiltration, a diagnosis of papillary squamous cell carcinoma in situ is adopted. These papillary tumours must be distinguished from squamous papilloma, transitional cell papilloma, inverted transitional cell papilloma, condyloma acuminatum with cytological atypia and verrucous carcinoma.

The infiltrating forms share the same prognosis as classic squamous cell carcinomas.

■ Lympho-epithelioma-like carcinoma [16, 29]

This is a tumour formation composed of undifferentiated uniform large cells with eosinophilic cytoplasm. The tumour cells combine syncytially; there is a stromal inflammatory infiltrate. On the periphery, this tumour formation appears sharply circumscribed; it is devoid of Epstein-Barr virus (EBV). The prognosis is better than in squamous cell carcinoma at the same stage (fewer nodal metastases). The differential diagnosis concerns glassy cell carcinoma and clearly circumscribed non-keratinising squamous carcinoma with marked inflammation.

The other tumour varieties are: spindle cell carcinoma (sarcomatoid carcinoma; squamous cell carcinoma with sarcoma-like stroma) and basaloid carcinoma (as in the ear nose and throat (ENT) region)

Adenocarcinoma *(table VIII)*

■ General remarks

Adenocarcinomas constitute 5% to 25% of carcinomas of the cervix. At present, an increasing frequency can be seen in both absolute and relative terms, particularly in young women (< 35 years). At the same time, there is a reduction in the frequency of squamous cell carcinomas. This is causing a variation in the ratio of adenocarcinomas/squamous cell carcinomas [25].

Pathogenically, adenocarcinomas of the cervix appear to relate both to squamous cell carcinomas of the cervix and adenocarcinomas of the endometrium. At least 50% of adenocarcinomas are associated with CIN or an infiltrating squamous cell carcinoma. HPV, particularly HPV 18, appears to be found in almost all adenocarcinomas. Other aetiological factors are common in adenocarcinomas of the uterine body: obesity,

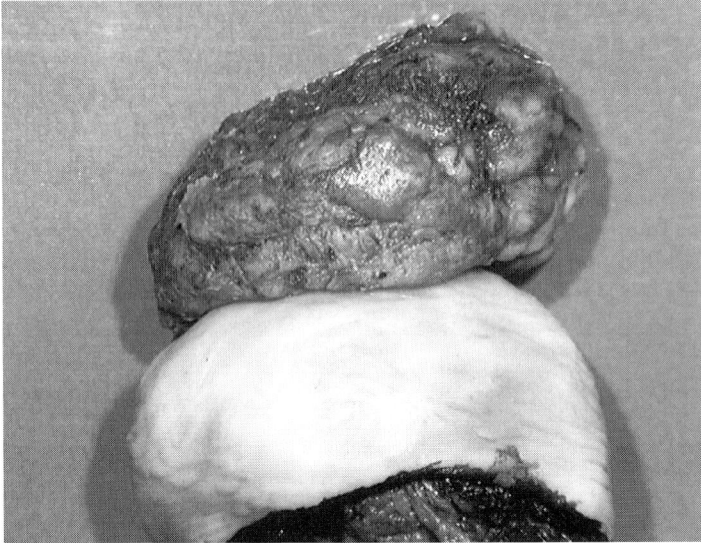

Figure 6. *Macroscopic aspect of an adenocarcinoma of the cervix. Its form is very polypoid.*

hypertension, diabetes, etc. The increase in the incidence of adenocarcinomas has cast suspicion on the role of prolonged, progestagen-rich oral contraception, but this is currently still a subject of dispute.

The mean age of onset is between 40 and 50 years, as with squamous cell carcinomas. However, adenocarcinomas might be more common in young women. Clinical features are present in 75% of cases, particularly vaginal bleeding.

Macroscopically almost half the cases appear polypoid, exophytic and papillary *(fig 6)*. In 15% of cases, the cervix is diffusely enlarged, nodular or ulcerated. In 15% of cases there is no macroscopic change. Even without this, the tumour may be deeply infiltrating. Cytological screening is possible in the majority of cases, but this is more difficult than with squamous cell carcinomas. Eighty-five percent of patients are stage I or II at the time of diagnosis.

Microscopically, glandular differentiation is observed. This microscopic appearance may vary according to the degree of differentiation, the type of adenocarcinoma, the extent of cytological atypia, mucosecretion, desmoplastic reaction, etc. The infiltrating component may be associated with a superficial papillary component, an adenocarcinoma in situ, CIN, etc. If several types of adenocarcinomas are present jointly, the classification is based on the predominant type, the other types being mentioned only if they constitute more than 10% of the tumour mass.

Problems of infiltration in adenocarcinomas

Adenocarcinoma does not infiltrate in the way that squamous cell carcinoma does. It may involve an infiltration in the form of glands. For this reason, the problems are different and often more difficult. A stromal desmoplastic reaction is not always present. A basement membrane may be found around the infiltrating glands. The diagnosis of infiltration is mainly based on the architecture and disposition of the glands. The normal glandular architecture is no longer maintained; glandular elements are found beneath the normal layer of glands (5 to 7 mm depth).

Micro-invasive adenocarcinoma is not currently deemed an individual entity. Any infiltrating lesion must be considered an infiltrating adenocarcinoma in its own right, even if the infiltration appears minimal [15].

Primary adenocarcinoma of the cervix versus extension into the cervix of an adenocarcinoma of the endometrium

An adenocarcinoma of the cervix derives in 50% of cases from a primary adenocarcinoma of the endocervix and in 50% from the spread to the cervix of an adenocarcinoma from the endometrium of the uterine corpus.

These two circumstances are difficult to distinguish morphologically. Mucinous type adenocarcinomas may also be observed in the endometrium. Endometroid type adenocarcinomas are the second most frequent type of tumour of the endocervix. Immunohistochemistry (CEA), which is particularly useful for defining the tumour type, cannot be used to determine the origin of the adenocarcinoma.

The differential diagnosis is based essentially on the clinical features and on examination of the hysterectomy specimen. An adenocarcinoma of the endometrium extending to the cervix has already infiltrated the uterine corpus and may be associated with atypical hyperplasia of the endometrium. Conversely, an adenocarcinoma of the endocervix tends to infiltrate the cervical wall extensively before spreading to the uterine corpus. It may be associated with CIN or adenocarcinoma in situ.

■ Conventional form - mucinous adenocarcinoma

This is the most frequent and the most common tumour variety and also the most indicative of an endocervical origin.

The glandular formations are lined with mucosecreting cells. This adenocarcinoma is usually highly or moderately differentiated. A peculiar pattern of growth is observed: abnormally crowded, with a complex branching acinar structure lacking the lobular architecture characteristic of normal endocervical glands. A "racemose" glandular pattern cribriform or papillary architecture may be observed.

In the intestinal forms, endocrine cells and Paneth cells may be found. Sometimes there are signet ring cells.

These tumours may be associated with mucinous tumours of the ovary.

The histochemical data (Alcian blue +, PAS +) and immunohistochemical data (carcinoembronic antigen) CEA +, vimentine -) contrast with those of endometrioid adenocarcinomas.

The differential diagnosis may include microglandular hyperplasia.

■ Endometrioid adenocarcinoma [2]

The appearance of this adenocarcinoma is entirely comparable to that of the most common form of adenocarcinomas of the endometrium (*fig 7*). This highlights from the outset the difficulty of a differential diagnosis with relation to the spread to the cervix of a poorly differentiated mucinous adenocarcinoma.

This adenocarcinoma may be associated with an endometrioid adenocarcinoma of the ovary.

■ Clear cell adenocarcinoma [20, 27]

Clear cell adenocarcinomas may occur at any age. Half to two-thirds of cases are related to exposure to DES. These cases are observed in particular in the youngest age

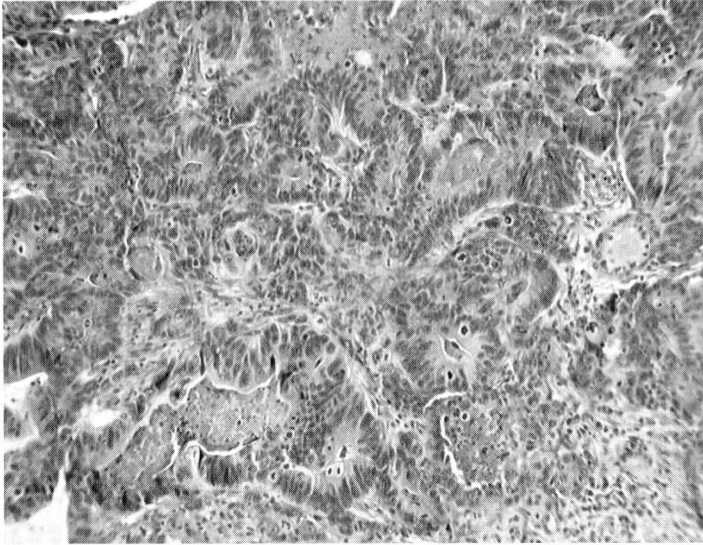

Figure 7. *Endometrioid adenocarcinoma (grade II).*

group (7 to 30 years) and a particularly short exposure may have been involved (1 week). In this context, this adenocarcinoma may be associated with other lesions: vaginal adenosis (50% of cases) or cervicovaginal abnormalities (20% of cases).

The histological appearance does not differ from that of the other clear cell adenocarcinomas. Several types of architecture may be observed: papillary, tubular, microcystic, solid. The tumour formations are lined with glycogen-rich "hobnail" clear cells *(fig 8)*. It should be noted that this tumour may sometimes be composed of eosinophilic rather than clear cells.

■ Serous adenocarcinoma [13, 30]

The histological appearance of this tumour does not differ in any way from that observed in serous adenocarcinomas of the endometrium, bladder, etc. This tumour is composed of papillary, often micropapillary, vegetations lined with particularly atypical cells.

This type of carcinoma is particularly aggressive: nodal metastases may be observed, even if the tumour appears relatively non-infiltrating.

This tumour must be distinguished from microglandular carcinomas.

■ Mesonephric adenocarcinoma

This type of tumour is exceptional. Several architectural forms may be observed: ductal, small tubular, retiform, solid, sex-cord, spindle.

Transitional images may be seen in neoplastic or hyperplastic mesonephric residues (sometimes florid and atypical hyperplasia).

This adenocarcinoma tends to be located deep in the vaginal wall under normal glandular mucosa. It should be noted that mesonephric residues are located on the lateral aspects of the cervical wall.

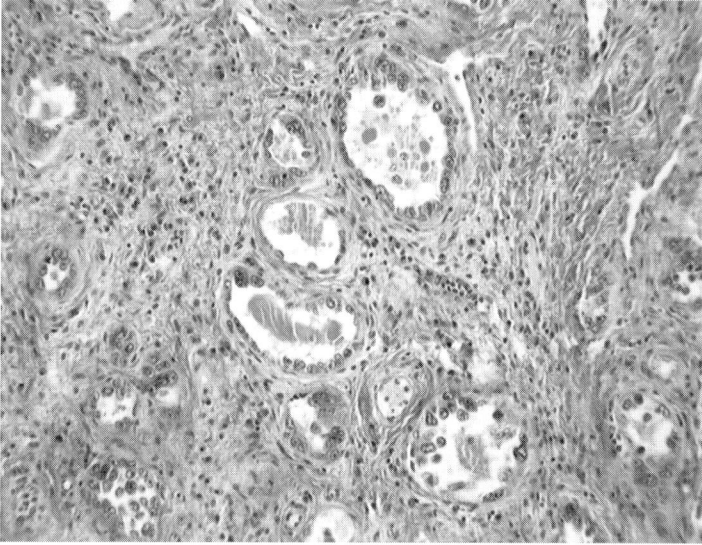

Figure 8. *Clear cell adenocarcinoma. Note the prominent nuclei and "hobnail" cells.*

■ Villoglandular adenocarcinoma [4, 12]

This is a well differentiated, polypoid, exophytic adenocarcinoma constituted essentially of arborescent papillary vegetations. These are long and thin (sometimes short and thick) and are lined with a cytologically non-atypical endocervical, endometrial or intestinal type epithelium (never by clear cell or serous epithelium). At the base of the lesion, it is possible to find an infiltrating component, more or less superficial and continuous with the papillary component. A fairly superficial invasion is usually involved.

This tumour variety occurs in younger women (35 to 40 years). The prognosis is good, with no metastatic spread. It may benefit from conservative treatment (conisation) if completely resected, the invasion is less than 3 mm and there is no vascular invasion.

■ Minimal deviation adenocarcinoma (MDA) or adenoma malignum [9]

This form of tumour (1% to 3% of adenocarcinomas) corresponds to a very highly differentiated adenocarcinoma both architecturally and cytologically. For this reason, diagnosis is particularly difficult, especially during initial biopsies. This explains the often belated diagnosis of this form of tumour at an advanced stage.

Several types of adenocarcinomas may exhibit this MDA appearance: the mucinous (the most common), endometrioid or clear cell types. The mucinous type may be observed in conjunction with Peutz-Jeghers syndrome. It may be associated with different types of ovarian tumours (mucinous tumours, sex cord-stromal tumours with annular tubules).

This adenocarcinomatous proliferation exhibits a characteristic growth pattern. Branching, irregularly oriented glands penetrate deep into the stroma and extend beyond the level of normal glands. The glands exhibit angular out-pouchings and complex outlines. Endocrine cells may be detected in the mucinous forms.

Traditionally, this form of tumour is associated with a poor prognosis. In reality, the prognosis is the same as for other types of adenocarcinomas at the same stage. The poor prognosis simply reflects the late diagnosis as a result of the initial diagnostic difficulties.

Problems of differential diagnosis may occur with several entities: endocervical tunnel clusters, deep lying cysts, endocervical adenomyoma, lobular endocervical glandular hyperplasia, etc. [11, 18].

Disease course and prognosis [21]

Spread is comparable to that of the squamous cell carcinomas. Local spread and distant nodal and visceral metastases appear earlier. After intracavitary treatment, it is more common to find a tumour residue than with squamous cell carcinomas.

Several parameters may affect the prognosis: stage, nodal metastases, tumour mass, depth of infiltration, vascular invasion, histological type, histological grade, aneuploidy, etc.

Globally, survival is lower than for squamous cell carcinomas. Global survival at 5 years is 48% to 56% (68% for squamous cell carcinomas).

Survival by stage is as follows:

– Stage 1: 84% (20% nodal metastases)

– Stage 2: 50%

– Stages 3, 4: 9%

Histological type does not have a major influence on the prognosis. The endometrioid type might have a better prognosis. The serous and clear cell types might have a more unfavourable prognosis, particularly those unrelated to DES.

Other epithelial tumours

■ Adenosquamous carcinoma

This is a tumour combining an adenocarcinomatous and a squamous carcinomatous component. The two components are usually poorly differentiated. The term adenosquamous carcinoma should only be used to describe:

– an squamous cell carcinoma of which some cells contain mucus, but without a glandular formation (muco-epidermoid carcinoma or variety of squamous cell carcinoma)

– an adenocarcinoma containing a cytologically benign squamous component (endometrioid adenocarcinoma with squamous metaplasia).

This tumour is primarily observed during pregnancy. The epidemiological risk factors are more similar to those of squamous cell carcinomas than those of adenocarcinoma.

The global prognosis is poorer than for the pure forms of squamous cell carcinoma or adenocarcinoma. However, no difference in prognosis is found at the same grades or stages.

■ Glassy cell carcinoma

This is a variant of undifferentiated adenocarcinoma or adenosquamous carcinoma: there is question of whether or not it is a true entity.

This tumour occurs in younger patients (mean age 40 years), sometimes during pregnancy.

The tumour cells are large. They have a "ground glass", granular, highly eosinophilic cytoplasm. The nuclei are also large with a prominent nucleolus. The cell membranes are clearly visible, particularly on PAS. There are abundant mitoses. The stroma may contain numerous inflammatory elements and in particular eosinophilic granulocytes. No very obvious squamous or glandular differentiation is found.

The prognosis is poor which might simply reflect the poor differentiation of the tumour.

■ Adenoid cystic carcinoma [3, 7, 22]

This tumour is observed in older patients (same age as for adenocarcinomas).

This tumour shows a fairly comparable histological appearance to that of other adenoid cystic carcinomas. Conversely, myo-epithelial cells are more difficult to visualise. This is usually a deeply infiltrating tumour, sometimes accompanied by lymphatic invasion. It may be associated with squamous metaplasia (60% of cases) or glandular neoplasia (16% of cases). Transitional features between adenoid cystic carcinoma and conventional adenocarcinoma may be observed.

This is a recurrent tumour which may produce bone or pulmonary metastases, etc.

The overall prognosis is poor, and worse than for squamous cell carcinomas. The prognosis is related to the stage; a number of deaths are observed at stage I.

It is a somewhat radio resistant tumour.

■ Adenoid basal carcinoma

This is a tumour that occurs in elderly women (mean age 60 years). There tend to be few signs and symptoms although there is sometimes an incidental finding in hysterectomy performed for other reasons.

Macroscopically, the changes are minor; the appearance is normal or there is a slight nodular distortion.

Microscopically there are nests and cords of small cells with peripheral palisading resembling basal cell carcinoma of the skin with squamous differentiation *(fig 9)*.

Squamous differentiation can occur; the presence of small glanduliform formations may be noted. Mitoses are rare. A desmoplastic stromal reaction is present in about 50% of cases. It should be noted that most nests produce no stromal reaction. This tumour may be fairly infiltrating locally and can be associated with CIN. The tumour is usually confined to the cervical region without metastatic spread.

■ Carcinoid tumour, small cell carcinoma, undifferentiated carcinoma [8]

A wide variety of names have been used to describe these tumours: argyrophilic carcinoma, neuro-endocrine carcinoma, poorly differentiated carcinoid, atypical carcinoid, apudoma.

Tumours with an endocrine differentiation exhibit a whole spectrum of differentiation. There is no truly typical carcinoid. The most well-differentiated tumours resemble the atypical carcinoid tumours. At the other end of the spectrum, there are small cell carcinomas. This endocrine differentiation may also be associated to squamous or glandular differentiation.

The most well-differentiated tumours have an organoid arrangement with a trabecular, insular, glandular and spindle pattern of growth. Small cell carcinomas resemble bronchial small cell carcinomas. There is a relationship between the degree of microscopic differentiation and clinical behaviour.

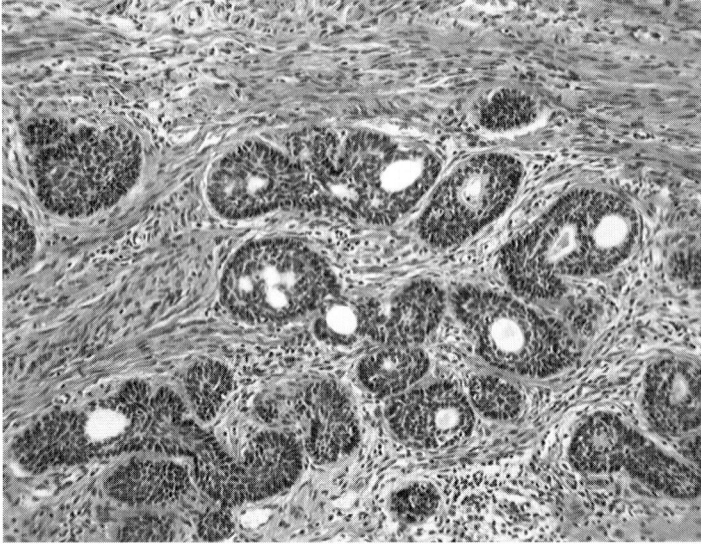

Figure 9. *Adenoid basal carcinoma. This tumour is made up of small nests of basaloid cells dug in glandular cavities.*

These tumours may present macroscopically in the form of an indurated lesion. They may be associated with HPV and produce different peptides.

These tumours must be distinguished from undifferentiated, non-keratinising, small cell squamous carcinomas and adenocarcinomas exhibiting carcinoid features.

Secondary tumours

■ Metastatic carcinoma

This is fairly rare and may be genital or extragenital in origin. In the cervix, they are more usually of genital origin (ovary, endometrium).

Metastases of extragenital origin are more common in the ovary or vagina. In the cervix the origin is primarily mammary and then gastro-intestinal.

Tumours of genital origin may involve migrant implants in the genital tract. Direct spread is also possible, particularly for tumours of endometrial, rectal or vesical origin. Fifty percent of adenocarcinomas of the cervix correspond to the spread to the cervix of an adenocarcinoma of endometrial origin.

Metastases may simulate a primary carcinoma of the cervix both clinically and histologically. They are rarely the principal features and a disseminated disease is already present in more than 90% of cases. Macroscopic spread is often minimal. An adenocarcinoma is usually involved (1% of adenocarcinomas of the cervix).

References

[1] Albores-Saavedra J, Gersell D, Gilks CB, Henson DE, Lindberg G, Santiago H et al. Terminology of endocrine tumors of the uterine cervix: results of a workshop sponsored by the College of American Pathologists and the National Cancer Institute. *Arch Pathol Lab Med* 1997 ; 121 : 34-39

[2] Alfsen GC, Thoresen SO, Kristensen GB, Skovlund E, Abeler VM. Histopathologic subtyping of cervical adenocarcinoma reveals increasing incidence rates of endometrioid tumors in all age groups: a population based study with review of all nonsquamous cervical carcinomas in Norway from 1966 to 1970, 1976 to 1980, and 1986 to 1990. *Cancer* 2000 ; 89 : 1291-1299

[3] Brainard JA, Hart WR. Adenoid basal epitheliomas of the uterine cervix: a reevaluation of distinctive cervical basaloid lesions currently classified as adenoid basal carcinoma and adenoid basal hyperplasia. *Am J Surg Pathol* 1998 ; 22 : 965-975

[4] Chang WC, Matisic JP, Zhou C, Thomson T, Clement PB, Hayes MM. Cytologic features of villoglandular adenocarcinoma of the uterine cervix: comparison with typical endocervical adenocarcinoma with a villoglandular component and papillary serous carcinoma. *Cancer* 1999 ; 87 : 5-11

[5] Creasman WT, Zaino RJ, Major FJ, Disaia PJ, Hatch KD, Homesley HD. Early invasive carcinoma of the cervix (3 to 5 mm invasion): risk factors and prognosis. A Gynecologic Oncology Group study. *Am J Obstet Gynecol* 1998 ; 178 (1 Pt 1) : 62-65

[6] Crum CP. Contemporary theories of cervical carcinogenesis: the virus, the host, and the stem cell. *Mod Pathol* 2000 ; 13 : 243-251

[7] Cviko A, Briem B, Granter SR, Pinto AP, Wang TY, Yang YC et al. Adenoid basal carcinomas of the cervix: a unique morphological evolution with cell cycle correlates. *Hum Pathol* 2000 ; 31 : 740-744

[8] Gilks CB, Young RH, Gersell DJ, Clement PB. Large cell neuroendocrine [corrected] carcinoma of the uterine cervix: a clinicopathologic study of 12 cases. *Am J Surg Pathol* 1997 ; 21 : 905-914

[9] Hayashi I, Tsuda H, Shimoda T. Reappraisal of orthodox histochemistry for the diagnosis of minimal deviation adenocarcinoma of the cervix. *Am J Surg Pathol* 2000 ; 24 : 559-562

[10] Huang CC, Kashima ML, Chen H, Shih IM, Kurman RJ, Wu TC. HPV in situ hybridization with catalyzed signal amplification and polymerase chain reaction in establishing cerebellar metastasis of a cervical carcinoma. *Hum Pathol* 1999 ; 30 : 587-591

[11] Jones MA, Young RH. Endocervical type A (noncystic) tunnel clusters with cytologic atypia. A report of 14 cases. *Am J Surg Pathol* 1996 ; 20 : 1312-1318

[12] Jones MW, Kounelis S, Papadaki H, Bakker A, Swalsky PA, Woods J et al. Well-differentiated villoglandular adenocarcinoma of the uterine cervix: oncogene/tumor suppressor gene alterations and human papillomavirus genotyping. *Int J Gynecol Pathol* 2000 ; 19 : 110-117

[13] Kaplan EJ, Caputo TA, Shen PU, Sassoon RI, Soslow RA. Familial papillary serous carcinoma of the cervix, peritoneum, and ovary: a report of the first case. *Gynecol Oncol* 1998 ; 70 : 289-294

[14] Kristensen GB, Abeler VM, Risberg B, Trop C, Bryne M. Tumor size, depth of invasion, and grading of the invasive tumor front are the main prognostic factors in early squamous cell cervical carcinoma. *Gynecol Oncol* 1999 ; 74 : 245-251

[15] Lee KR, Flynn CE. Early invasive adenocarcinoma of the cervix. *Cancer* 2000 ; 89 : 1048-1055

[16] Lopez-Rios F, Miguel PS, Bellas C, Ballestin C, Hernandez L. Lymphoepithelioma-like carcinoma of the uterine cervix: a case report studied by in situ hybridization and polymerase chain reaction for Epstein-Barr virus. *Arch Pathol Lab Med* 2000 ; 124 : 746-747

[17] Mannion C, Park WS, Man YG, Zhuang Z, Albores-Saavedra J, Tavassoli FA. Endocrine tumors of the cervix: morphologic assessment, expression of human papillomavirus, and evaluation for loss of heterozygosity on 1p, 3p, 11q, and 17p. *Cancer* 1998 ; 83 : 1391-1400

[18] Nucci MR, Clement PB, Young RH. Lobular endocervical glandular hyperplasia, not otherwise specified: a clinicopathologic analysis of thirteen cases of a distinctive pseudoneoplastic lesion and comparison with fourteen cases of adenoma malignum. *Am J Surg Pathol* 1999 ; 23 : 886-891

[19] Ostor AG. Early invasive adenocarcinoma of the uterine cervix. *Int J Gynecol Pathol* 2000 ; 19 : 29-38

[20] Reich O, Tamussino K, Lahousen M, Pickel H, Haas J, Winter R. Clear cell carcinoma of the uterine cervix: pathology and prognosis in surgically treated stage IB-IIB disease in women not exposed in utero to diethylstilbestrol. *Gynecol Oncol* 2000 ; 76 : 331-335

[21] Sakuragi N, Takeda N, Hareyama H, Fujimoto T, Todo Y, Okamoto K et al. A multivariate analysis of blood vessel and lymph vessel invasion as predictors of ovarian and lymph node metastases in patients with cervical carcinoma. *Cancer* 2000 ; 88 : 2578-2583

[22] Samaratunga H. Cervical adenoid basal epitheliomas. *Am J Surg Pathol* 1999 ; 23 : 1308-1309

[23] Sasagawa T, Shimakage M, Nakamura M, Sakaike J, Ishikawa H, Inoue M. Epstein-Barr virus (EBV) genes expression in cervical intraepithelial neoplasia and invasive cervical cancer: a comparative study with human papillomavirus (HPV) infection. *Hum Pathol* 2000 ; 31 : 318-326

[24] Skyldberg B, Salo S, Eriksson E, Aspenblad U, Moberger B, Tryggvason K et al. Laminin-5 as a marker of invasiveness in cervical lesions. *J Natl Cancer Inst* 1999 ; 91 : 1882-1887

[25] Smith HO, Tiffany MF, Qualls CR, Key CR. The rising incidence of adenocarcinoma relative to squamous cell carcinoma of the uterine cervix in the United States--a 24-year population-based study. *Gynecol Oncol* 2000 ; 78 : 97-105

[26] Suen KC. Cytological recognition of invasive squamous cancer of the uterine cervix. *Hum Pathol* 2000 ; 31 : 774-775

[27] Tambouret R, Bell DA, Young RH. Microcystic endocervical adenocarcinomas: a report of eight cases. *Am J Surg Pathol* 2000 ; 24 : 369-374

[28] Trivijitsilp P, Mosher R, Sheets EE, Sun D, Crum CP. Papillary immature metaplasia (immature condyloma) of the cervix: a clinicopathologic analysis and comparison with papillary squamous carcinoma. *Hum Pathol* 1998 ; 29 : 641-648

[29] Tseng CJ, Pao CC, Tseng LH, Chang CT, Lai CH, Soong YK et al. Lymphoepithelioma-like carcinoma of the uterine cervix: association with Epstein-Barr virus and human papillomavirus. *Cancer* 1997 ; 80 : 91-97

[30] Zhou C, Gilks CB, Hayes M, Clement PB. Papillary serous carcinoma of the uterine cervix: a clinicopathologic study of 17 cases. *Am J Surg Pathol* 1998 ; 22 : 113-120

Chapter 5

Staging and pretherapeutic investigations

Carlos De Oliveira, Fernando Mota

C De Oliveira, *Professor of Gynaecology, Head of Department of Gynaecological Oncology.*
F Mota, *Auxiliary Professor of Gynaecology.*
University Hospital of Coimbra, 3049 Coimbra, Portugal.

Staging and pretherapeutic investigations

C De Oliveira, F Mota

Abstract. — An overview on the staging of carcinoma of the cervix uteri is presented. The importance of a clinical examination under anaesthesia is emphasised. The complementary procedures and accepted auxiliary examinations for cancer staging are analysed. A summarised description of the optional investigations that can improve clinical staging is also presented. It is stressed that cervical cancer staging does not limit treatment strategies which must be tailored to the disease on an individual basis.

Keywords: clinical examination, CT scan, cystoscopy, intravenous pyelogram, lymphangiography, rectosigmoidoscopy, staging, ultrasonography.

Introduction

Accurate cervical cancer staging (assessing the extent of the disease) is necessary for the selection of appropriate treatment modalities and for planning their sequence. Staging is also important, not only as a means of evaluating treatment strategies within one institution, but also because it provides a means of comparing results from different institutions throughout the world. It should therefore be done as uniformly as possible. Accurate staging is also essential in optimising the results of therapy, because therapy and prognosis vary considerably from stage to stage. However, staging does not limit treatment modalities, and therapy can be tailored to the architecture of the tumour in each patient.

Clinical staging

It is agreed that staging of cervical cancer is a predominantly clinical process, preferably with the patient anaesthetised. It cannot be changed later if findings at operation or subsequent treatment reveal further disease, since this "upstaging" of patients would produce erroneous improvements in the results of treatment of early-stage disease. The pretherapeutic investigations that can be used for staging cervical cancer are presented *(table I)*.

■ Clinical examination and complementary procedures

The great majority of patients will have a normal general physical examination. However, the inguinal lymph nodes should be palpated, particularly if the lower third of the vagina has been invaded. Supraclavicular lymph nodes should also be palpated since they can be the site of distant metastases, even in apparently early-stage cervical cancers. Abdominal palpation is carried out to look for ascites or hepatomegaly. The aetiology of a pleural effusion or a swollen leg is investigated. All these conditions may be evidence of metastatic disease.

Table I. Pretherapeutic investigations.

Clinical examination	General physical examination Genital examination Bimanual rectovaginal examination (under anaesthesia)
Procedures	Colposcopy Biopsy Endocervical curettage Conisation
Auxiliary examinations	Intravenous pyelogram Cystoscopy Rectosigmoidoscopy Chest X-ray Skeletal X-ray
Optional investigations	Lymphangiography Computerised axial tomography Ultrasonography Magnetic resonance imaging Radionucleotide scanning Laparoscopy

Examination of the vulva and perineum may rarely identify an in situ or cancerous lesion. The relationship between the urethral orifice and an eventual lesion in the lower third of the vagina is recorded. All suspicious lesions should be biopsied to confirm the diagnosis of metastases.

At speculum examination, the cervix may appear entirely normal if the cancer is very small (subclinical) or located in the endocervix. For patients with suspected early invasive cancer based on Papanicolaou (Pap) test results and a normal-appearing cervix, colposcopy is mandatory and will identify the most suspicious area to be biopsied. Colposcopic findings suggestive of early cervical cancer are: atypical blood vessels (abnormal in size, shape, calibre, direction), irregular surface contours, an ulcerated, friable and yellow-orange epithelium, large and severe or complex colposcopic abnormalities, and their extension into the canal.

The incidence of cervical adenocarcinomas is increasing, accounting for about 20% of cervical neoplasms. Sometimes the adenocarcinoma appears as a papillary lesion on the portio. However, it generally develops within the canal when the ectocervix appears totally normal, at least initially. In these circumstances, an endocervical curettage is mandatory as the final step of a careful colposcopic examination.

Punch biopsies are adequate for the confirmation of a clinically obvious cancer. However, if the diagnosis cannot be established conclusively with biopsy or endocervical curettage, diagnostic conisation is necessary. Furthermore, punch biopsies are not sufficient for the definitive diagnosis of microinvasive cervical cancer and again a conisation is indicated to correctly assess the depth and horizontal extent of microinvasion involvement as well as vascular penetration.

The lesion on the ectocervix can be exophytic with a cauliflower-like appearance; irregular; variable in size; sometimes with a firm, elevated margin; and haemorrhagic. The lesion can also be ulcerated with an indurated base, in which case the cervix and eventually the vaginal fornices may be replaced by a necrotic crater. Sometimes an infiltrating tumour shows a little visible ulceration or exophytic mass but it is perceived as a stone-hard cervix on palpation. As the tumour develops, a gross cervix may be found (the so-called "barrel-shaped cervix") when a squamous cell carcinoma involves the whole cervix or an infiltrative endocervical tumour develops inside the canal. After examination of the cervix, the vaginal walls and particularly the vaginal fornices are carefully inspected to look for suspicious lesions. Biopsies should be performed.

■ Pelvic examination under anaesthesia

This step of the evaluation, carried out by at least one, generally two, experienced oncologists, is fundamental for the staging of cervical cancer since the true extent of the cancer may be underestimated if rectovaginal examination under anaesthesia is omitted. This examination is indispensable for evaluating the extension of the tumour towards the vaginal fornices, down the vagina, laterally into the parametria, anteriorly into the vesicovaginal space, or posteriorly into the uterosacral ligaments. Vaginal palpation will specify tumour volume, as well as the size and consistency of the cervix. Endophytic or infiltrative cervical cancers can be suspected due to a stone-hard consistency of the cervix upon palpation. Infiltrative vaginal lesions can also be detected during this procedure, but are often missed during vaginal inspection.

Transrectal palpation under anaesthesia is indispensable in evaluating the parametria:

– Are they soft/elastic, or nodular and invaded by the tumour? The tumour is often secondarily infected. It is, therefore, sometimes impossible to know how much of the fixation and thickening in the parametria are due to tumour or to inflammatory reaction. Preliminary antibiotic and anti-inflammatory treatment can be prescribed.

– Is the invasion unilateral or bilateral?

– Is there tissue fixation onto the pelvic wall? Sometimes a nodular/invaded uterosacral ligament can be felt. An enlarged pelvic lymph node can be palpated. The gynaecologist will evaluate softness and mobility or invasion of the rectum. The eventual invasion of the rectovaginal space can also be detected by inserting the index finger into the vagina and the middle finger into the rectum.

Laboratory investigations

A general biological evaluation using clinical as well as an array of laboratory tests is performed in order to evaluate patient general health, and any metabolic, renal or cardiorespiratory functions which may contraindicate surgery. In addition, haemoglobin levels should be determined and anaemia corrected. Abnormal liver function tests may indicate metastases in this organ. Hypercalcemia may denote advanced disease with bone involvement.

The tumour marker SCC ("squamous cell carcinoma") should be determined prior to any therapy and if elevated, may be a useful marker in assessing response to therapy. Increased serum levels are found in 50% to 75% of locally advanced cancers, and the titer value correlates to stage, tumour volume and prognosis. In adenocarcinomas of the cervix, preoperative measurement of the tumour marker CA125 should be obtained.

Auxiliary examinations for staging

The necessary procedures for staging cervical cancer and the acceptable auxiliary examinations to improve clinical evaluation are listed *(table I)*. Optional investigations, the information from which is not allowed by FIGO to change the clinical stage, are also presented. The findings of the optional investigations are not used in assigning the FIGO stage because the techniques involved are not uniformly available throughout the world, and interpretation of their results is variable. However, the information provided by these optional investigations may be used in planning therapy.

■ Intravenous pyelogram

This examination is frequently normal. However, double ureters can be found and their position determined which is of utmost importance during surgery. The finding of a pelvic kidney must be taken into account when delineating the pelvic fields for radiotherapy. Abnormalities can sometimes be found involving the ureters, bladder or kidneys, particularly in advanced cervical cancers. Any deviation, angulation, rigidity or obstruction of the ureters should be recorded, since they may be directly invaded by the regional spread of the tumour (especially in the vicinity of the bladder), or an adenopathy may compress or deviate them.

Hydronephrosis, secretion retardation or a non-functioning kidney may be present. The bladder may show an encroachment evoking compression, or an irregularity and/or rigidity suggesting invasion by the tumour.

■ Cystoscopy

Cystoscopy is seldom productive in evaluating stage I and II cervical cancer patients. However, this examination is helpful in defining the integrity/invasion of the bladder.

Careful inspection of the mucosa of the bladder, as well as trigone and ureter orifices should be undertaken. A normal, pink bladder mucosa may be the site of erythema or leucoplasia. Single or multiple exophytic growths, granulations, ulcerations, and localised oedema may all be hallmarks of invasion of the bladder mucosa. Biopsies of these suspicious areas are necessary in confirming the diagnosis. It should be remembered, though, that submucosal invasion of the bladder may be missed by cystoscopy.

■ Rectosigmoidoscopy

This is useful only when the tumour invades posteriorly and the rectovaginal space is infiltrated. It allows the observation of rectal and lower colon mucosae that may be normal or congestive, fixed, showing friable and bloody vegetations, or its lumen may be stenosed by extension of the cervical tumour to the muscularis layer. Biopsies should be performed.

■ Chest X-ray (posteroanterior and lateral)

Although pulmonary metastases are uncommon, they need to be ruled out. In advanced disease, lung metastases are present in approximately 5% of cases that would otherwise be stage III or IVa. Chest X-ray is also useful to the anaesthetist for evaluating the cardiorespiratory status of the patient.

■ Skeletal X-ray

This examination is unproductive because bone metastases are rare and frequently symptomatic.

The FIGO staging system

The current staging system of the International Federation of Gynaecology and Obstetrics (FIGO) for cervical carcinoma is presented [5] *(table II)*. This classification applies only to carcinoma, and there should be histological confirmation of the disease. When there is doubt in deciding on a stage, the earlier stage should be chosen. The diagnosis of both stages Ia1 and Ia2 should be based on microscopic examination of removed tissue, preferably a cone, which must include the entire lesion. The depth of invasion should not be more than 5 mm taken from the base of the epithelium, either surface or glandular, from which it originates to the deepest point of invasion. The second dimension, the horizontal spread, must not exceed 7 mm. Vascular space involvement, either venous or lymphatic, should not alter the staging, but should be recorded as it may affect future treatment decisions. Lesions of greater size should be staged as Ib. As a rule, it is impossible to estimate clinically whether a cancer of the cervix has extended to the corpus. Extension to the corpus should therefore be disregarded.

Some authors support the subdivision of stage Ia into "early stromal invasion" (i.e. microscopic epithelial neoplastic buds which emanate from the base of a carcinoma in situ), and "microinvasion" to a depth of between 1 and 5 mm. It is argued that there is a significant difference in terms of recurrence, vascular invasion, and survival between the two histopathological entities [3]. The purpose of this classification is to identify a group of patients who are not at risk for lymph node metastases or recurrence and who may be treated conservatively.

Table II. FIGO staging of carcinoma of the cervix uteri.

Pre-invasive Carcinoma

Stage 0 — Carcinoma in situ, intraepithelial carcinoma (these cases should not be included in any therapeutic statistics).

Invasive Carcinoma

Stage I — Carcinoma strictly confined to the cervix (textension to the corpus should be disregarded).

    Stage Ia — Pre-clinical carcinomas, i.e. those diagnosed only by microscopy.

        Stage Ia1 Lesions with ≤ 3 mm invasion.

        Stage Ia2 Lesions detected microscopically that can be measured. Depth of invasion of > 3 to 5 mm. Horizontal spread must not exceed 7 mm.

    Stage Ib — Lesions invasive > 5 mm.

        Stage Ib1 Lesions ≤ 4 cm.

        Stage Ib2 Lesions > 4 cm.

Stage II — Carcinoma extends beyond the cervix but not onto the pelvic wall. Carcinoma involves the vagina, but not the lower third.

    Stage IIa No obvious parametrial involvement.

    Stage IIb Obvious parametrial involvement.

Stage III — Carcinoma has extended onto the pelvic wall. On rectal examination, there is no cancer-free space between the tumour and the pelvic wall. The tumour involves the lower third of the vagina. All cases with hydronephrosis or non-functioning kidney (unless known to be due to another cause).

    Stage IIIa No extension to the pelvic wall.

    Stage IIIb Extension onto the pelvic wall and/or hydronephrosis or non-functioning kidney.

Stage IV — Carcinoma has extended beyond the true pelvis or has clinically involved the mucosa of the bladder or rectum.

    Stage IVa Spread of the tumour to adjacent organs.

    Stage IVb Spread to distant organs.

A patient with a tumour fixed to the pelvic wall by a short and indurated but not nodular parametrium should be assigned to stage IIb. On clinical examination, it is impossible to decide whether a smooth, indurated parametrium is truly cancerous or only inflammatory. Therefore, the case should be assigned to stage III only if the parametrium is nodular to the pelvic wall or the tumour itself extends to the pelvic wall. The presence of hydronephrosis or a non-functioning kidney, due to stenosis of the ureter by cancer, means that a case is allotted to stage III even if, according to other findings, it should be assigned to stage I or II.

The presence of a bullous oedema, as such, should not permit a case to be assigned to stage IV. Ridges and furrows in the bladder wall should be interpreted as signs of submucous involvement of the bladder if they remain fixed to the tumour on palpation (i.e. examination from the vagina or the rectum during cystoscopy). Finally, a cytological finding of malignant cells in washings from the bladder requires further examination and a biopsy specimen from the mucosa of the bladder.

Optional investigations

It is obvious that none of the previously described procedures and techniques yields information on the commonest metastatic pathway of cervical cancer: the lymphatic system. Knowledge of lymph node status, among others, is useful in devising a therapeutic programme for the patient. Thus, lymphangiography, ultrasonography, and, more recently, computerised axial tomography, magnetic resonance imaging, and even fine-needle lymph node aspiration are employed.

It must be emphasised that the results of these investigations will not change the patient's reported stage, but may change her treatment, i.e. an individualised treatment programme, appropriate to the patient's stage and disease. Furthermore, the results of the imaging modalities highlight the limitations of the clinical staging.

■ Lymphangiography

Since lymphangiography is the only examination where the internal architecture of the lymph nodes will be observed, it is, at least theoretically, very important, but it causes some controversy. It is a fairly difficult study, has low sensitivity although excellent specificity, and its role in the future management of patients with cervical cancer is questionable for some oncologists. Sensitivity is lowest with small metastases, and even large nodal deposits can be missed.

A radiotransparent image in an enlarged node is particularly suggestive of nodal invasion, as are blockage or asymmetry of pelvic and para-aortic lymph nodes [11]. Piver et al [12] reported that lymphangiography can detect 78% of histopathologically documented lymph node invasion. Fuchs and Rosenberg [7] showed 87% accurate diagnoses, with 1.5% false positive and 12% false negative results. The main factors that contribute to these rates are: the congenital absence of some lymph nodes, some pelvic and para-aortic nodes are not opacified, inflammation and the size of the metastases (they need to be 5 to 10 mm in diameter to be visible [6]). Tuberculosis or endometriosis can also induce false positive results. Lymphangiography has its merits, however. It has been shown to be of prognostic value in stage III. The overall 5 year survival rate was 58% versus 17%, comparing negative and positive lymphangiographic findings [7]. Similar conclusions were reported by Hammond et al [8] for cervical cancers in stages Ib to IIIb. Moreover, suspect para-aortic nodes can be sampled during surgery, or radiotherapeutic fields extended to involve these areas.

■ Computerised axial tomography (CT scan)

Parametrial (especially its inner third) and vaginal invasion are often undetected. False positive results are also common, since it is difficult to differentiate invasion from inflammation, prior radiation or infection [19]. In contrast, CT scan in advanced cervical cancer (stages IIb to IV) seems capable of improving clinical findings by defining the tumour volume accurately, evaluating adjacent structures for contiguous involvement and also allowing the study of the liver and urinary system [6]. A recent study has shown the positive predictive value of CT scan in predicting bladder invasion to be 60%, with a negative predictive value of 100% [17]. CT scan can allow direct visualisation of the ureters, retroperitoneum, pelvic sidewalls, and adenopathies. The bowel can be opacified and vascular structures enhanced with contrast. For all these reasons, CT scan is of value in monitoring therapy.

Although it cannot detect invasion of normal sized lymph nodes, especially pelvic nodes, this technique has a fair specificity and sensitivity (about 70% to 80%) in identifying abnormal para-aortic lymph nodes [2, 6]. Optimally, positive nodes should be documented by fine-needle aspiration or surgical excision because the CT scan has a 5% to 10% false positive rate [1].

■ Ultrasonography

The genito-urinary and the lymphatic systems can be explored by this technique. It is also useful for patients with leg oedema, in differentiating lymphatic obstruction from deep vein thrombosis. The current use of transvaginal and/or transrectal probes has considerably increased the sensitivity of ultrasonography when evaluating tumour volume and its local spread (parametria, bladder), and can be used to monitor treatment. In addition, hydronephrosis may not only be detected but also followed up during radiotherapy. The sensitivity of ultrasonography is, however, lower than that of lymphangiography and CT scan in detecting lymph nodes. Sonography is also operator-dependent, and is unlikely to give objective and reproducible data for tumour classification.

■ Magnetic resonance imaging (MRI)

MRI seems promising in evaluating parametrial involvement, with a sensitivity of 85% to 92%. Its sensitivity in evaluating the vesicovaginal space has been reported to be between 75% and 85% [6]. Precise measurements of cervical tumours (depth of stromal invasion and tumour volume), and therapy monitoring are obtained particularly in advanced stages, but also in stage Ib [15]. Even high resolution MRI for diagnosis of invaded pelvic lymph nodes has been reported to have only a 68% sensitivity and 78% specificity [9].

■ Comparison of optional investigations

Compared to MRI, CT scan permits effective visualisation of the thorax and upper abdomen. Another advantage of CT scan over MRI is the availability of bowel contrast and visualisation of the urinary tract and hepatic metastases. Unlike MRI, CT scan and sonography-guided fine needle aspiration biopsy provide a means of studying the nature of a suspect lesion located in the parametrium or lymph nodes and of confirming tumour recurrence. However, MRI has a greater capacity than CT scan to discriminate between cancer and normal cervical and uterine tissue. Hence, MRI is more useful in the design of optimal radiation treatment portals.

To evaluate tumour volume, parametrial and vesicovaginal extension, MRI is superior to CT scan and sonography, both in pretherapeutic investigation and in follow-up assessment [4, 6]. It is generally accepted that nodal involvement is better evaluated by lymphography followed by CT scan. However, the results of a recent meta-analysis showed no statistically significant difference comparing lymphography, CT scan and MRI in the evaluation of lymph node metastases [16]. When a recurrence is suspected, a CT scan should be performed. Eventually, as a second-line examination, MRI may also help to differentiate between fibrosis and relapse of disease.

■ Laparoscopy

Considering the discordance ranging from 30% to 70% between clinical staging and findings during surgery [18, 20], laparoscopy can improve cervical cancer staging. Unsuspected or inconspicuous intraperitoneal, adnexal or liver metastases may be diagnosed. Intraperitoneal biopsies and washings can be carried out and discriminate between inflammation and invasion. Moreover, laparoscopic evaluation and sampling of pelvic and para-aortic lymph nodes have been reported to have a sensitivity and specificity of about 92% in identifying disease [14] and this may change the primary therapy offered to the patient.

Surgical and pathological staging

Some factors (e.g. absence or presence and level of lymph node metastases, or subclinical parametrial extension) which have prognostic significance and affect the selection and sequencing of treatment modalities are not taken into account in clinical staging.

Surgical staging of patients with cervical cancer shows that a proportion have extrapelvic lymph node metastases lying outside conventional radiation fields. Treatment with extended volume radiation fields can result in salvaging some of these patients [13]. However, surgical staging may delay initiation of radiation and increase treatment complications (e.g. deep vein thrombosis, pulmonary embolus, bowel obstruction). Furthermore, the novel and more accurate imaging techniques can spare cervical cancer patients the potential morbidity and mortality of surgical staging.

After surgery, the pathological findings in the removed specimens can form the basis for very precise evaluation of the extent of the disease: pathological staging. These findings should not alter the clinical staging but should be recorded, to help management of the patient and as valuable prognostic parameters.

References

[1] Bandy LC, Clarke-Pearson DL, Silverman PM, Creasman WT. Computed tomography in evaluation of extrapelvic lymphadenectomy in carcinoma of the cervix. *Obstet Gynecol* 1985 ; 65 : 73-76

[2] Brenner DE, Whitley NO, Prempree T, Villasanta U. An evaluation of the computed tomographic scanner for the staging of carcinoma of the cervix. *Cancer* 1982 ; 50 : 2323-2328

[3] Burghardt E, Östör A, Fox H. The new FIGO definition of cervical cancer stage IA: a critique. *Gynecol Oncol* 1997 ; 65 : 1-5

[4] Cobby M, Browning J, Jones A, Whipp E, Goddard P. Magnetic resonance imaging, computed tomography and endosonography in the local staging of carcinoma of the cervix. *Br J Radiol* 1990 ; 63 : 673-679

[5] Creasman WT. New gynecologic cancer staging. *Gynecol Oncol* 1995 ; 58 : 157-158

[6] Darbois Y, Buthiau D, Dargent D. Cancer du col utérin. In : Buthiau D, Khayat D eds. Scanner et IRM en cancérologie. Berlin : Springer-Verlag, 1995 : 279-290

[7] Fuchs WA, Rosenberg GS. Lymphography in carcinoma of the uterine cervix. *Acta Radiol* 1975 ; 16 : 353-361

[8] Hammond JA, Herson J, Freedman RS, Hamberger AD, Wharton JT, Wallace S et al. The impact of lymph node status on survival in cervical carcinoma. *Int J Radiat Oncol Biol Phys* 1981 ; 7 : 1713-1718

[9] Hawighorst H, Schoenberg SO, Knapstein PG, Knopp MV, Schaeffer U, Essig M et al. Staging of invasive cervical carcinoma and of pelvic lymph nodes by high resolution MRI with a phased-array coil in comparison with pathological findings. *J Comput Assist Tomogr* 1998 ; 22 : 75-81

[10] Koelher PR, Wohl GT, Schaffer B. Lymphangiography. A survey of its current status. *AJR Am J Roentgenol* 1964 ; 91 : 1216-1223

[11] Leman MH Jr, Park RC, Barham ED, Chism SE, Petty WM, Patow WE. Pretreatment lymphangiography in carcinoma of the uterine cervix. *Gynecol Oncol* 1975 ; 3 : 354-360

[12] Piver MS, Wallace S, Castro JR. The accuracy of lymphangiography in carcinoma of the uterine cervix. *AJR Am J Roentgenol* 1971 ; 111 : 278-283

[13] Podczaski E, Stryker JA, Kaminski P, Ndubisi B, Larson J, Degeest K et al. Extended-field radiation therapy for carcinoma of the cervix. *Cancer* 1990 ; 66 : 251-258

[14] Possover M, Krause N, Kuhne-Heid R, Schneider A. Value of laparoscopic evaluation of para-aortic and pelvic lymph nodes for treatment of cervical cancer. *Am J Obs Gynecol* 1998 ; 178 : 806-810

[15] Rubens D, Thornbury JR, Angel C, Stoler MH, Weiss SL, Lerner RM et al. Stage IB cervical carcinoma: comparison of clinical, MR, and pathologic staging. *AJR Am J Roentgenol* 1988 ; 150 : 135-138

[16] Scheidler J, Hricak H, Yu KK, Subak L, Segal MR. Radiological evaluation of lymph node metastases in patients with cervical cancer. A meta-analysis. *JAMA* 1997 ; 278 : 1096-1101

[17] Sundborg MJ, Taylor RR, Mark J, Elg SA. Cystoscopy after computed tomography scan to identify bladder invasion in cervical cancer. *Obstet Gynecol* 1998 ; 92 : 364-366

[18] Twiggs LB, Potish RA, George RJ, Adcock LL. Pretreatment extraperitoneal surgical staging in primary carcinoma of the cervix uteri. *Surg Gynecol Obstet* 1984 ; 158 : 243-250

[19] Villasanta V, Whittley NO, Haney PJ, Brenner D. Computed tomography in invasive carcinoma of the cervix: an appraisal. *Obstet Gynecol* 1983 ; 62 : 218-224

[20] Wharton JT, Jones HW, Day TG Jr, Rutledge FN, Fletcher GH. Pre-irradiation celiotomy and extended field irradiation for invasive carcinoma of the cervix. *Obstet Gynecol* 1977 ; 49 : 333-338

Chapter 6

Treatment of micro-invasive cervical carcinoma

Péter Bösze

P Bösze, M.D., Ph.D., D.Sc., Professor and Chairman, European Academy of Gynaecological Cancer, EAGC, International Institute of Cancer Genetics, Department of Gynaecology, Saint Stephen Hospital, Nagyvárad tér 1, 1096 Budapest, Hungary.

Treatment of micro-invasive cervical carcinoma

Péter Bösze

Abstract. — *The definition and treatment of micro-invasive cervical carcinoma are still debated. The quantified current International Federation of Gynecology and Obstetrics (FIGO) staging provides a ground for further studies. The ideal definition of micro-invasive cervical carcinoma should involve evidence-based predictive factors, in addition to the anatomical description of the disease extension, i.e. stage. Much is settled in the management of stage IA1 lesions, and fortunately, the majority of women with micro-invasive disease belong to this group. As for stage IA2 lesions, the true incidence of extra-uterine involvement and the recurrence rate have yet to be determined. What may guide the gynaecological oncologist in treating this neoplasm is the evaluation of as many conventional and molecular prognostic factors as available, including true depth and width of invasion irrespective of categories, i.e. from the FIGO staging. The more superficial the invasion, the lower the risk of spread of the disease outside the cervix: e.g. a lesion with 1 mm depth of invasion is practically never associated with extra-cervical metastasis. The significance of horizontal spread has not been well appreciated. The prognostic value of lymphatic or vascular space involvement (LVSI) is controversial. The pathologist plays a vital role in the management, and appropriate histological evaluation of the cone specimen is a prerequisite of any therapy. Stage IA1 lesions can be safely treated with therapeutic conisation provided the margins are free of atypical cells. Hysterectomy is recommended only in the presence of additional indications. Management of stage IA2 squamous cell lesions continues to be debated. For local control, conisation or simple hysterectomy, the latter mostly in the presence of additional indications, including postmenopausal age, are adequate. There is no convincing evidence for the use of modified or extended radical hysterectomy although it may be indicated in the presence of positive pelvic nodes. In spite of this, a modified radical hysterectomy has been recommended and is being used in many centres worldwide. Radical vaginal trachelectomy is a valuable alternative to modified radical hysterectomy in high-risk patients when childbearing is of concern. Pelvic lymphadenectomy is recommended but has not been substantiated as a standard procedure and should be tailored to risk factors.*

Keywords: micro-invasive cervical carcinoma, treatment, follow-up.

Introduction

The definition of micro-invasive cervical carcinoma has evolved over the last decades and undergone several changes. The current FIGO definition was established in 1994. Accordingly, stage IA1 cancer includes lesions with 0-3 mm invasion in depth and not exceeding 7 mm in width. Stage IA2 has 3-5 mm of invasion, limited to 7 mm in width. Lymphatic or vascular space involvement (LVSI) should not alter the staging. All large lesions, even with superficial invasions, are stage IB cancer [4]. Whether it is an ideal definition of micro-invasive disease for guiding therapy remains to be determined. It should be noted that 1) micro-invasive cervical carcinoma is surgically staged, in contrast to other cervical carcinomas that are clinically staged; 2) approximately 20% of microscopic cervical carcinoma is not classified as micro-invasive because it is over the 7 mm width limit.

In early reports, micro-invasive carcinoma constituted only 2% to 8% of invasive cervical carcinomas. With the introduction of more effective screening, its incidence is steadily increasing. Studies have reported incidences of up to 25% [14]. This increase in micro-invasive carcinoma puts emphasis on the future clinical impact of this early neoplastic disease. Approximately 60% to 70% of patients have stage IA1 disease, the majority having lesions with invasion of less than 1 mm in depth [9].

The diagnosis of micro-invasive carcinoma is made histologically and requires a conisation specimen with clear margins in all directions, such as cervical, endocervical and deep margins, to study the entire lesion. Early invasion mostly originates from carcinoma in situ; in rare cases, however, only lower-grade cervical intrepithelial neoplasia (CIN) is present. The invasion involves multiple points in a substantial number of cases, making histological work-up difficult. A histological description of the lesions is beyond the scope of this chapter. In the absence of tumour-free (including CIN-free) margins, adequate staging is not possible. Evaluation of the margins may occasionally be difficult due to the thermal effect of laser or diathermy surgery. A thin lesion-free margin may be destroyed and erroneously diagnosed as a positive margin, i.e. a false positive margin. Screening cytology has been reported to be very accurate (60-80%) in predicting squamous cell micro-invasive carcinoma [14].

The histological criteria of squamous cell micro-invasive cervical carcinoma are the depth of invasion (up to 5 mm) and the horizontal extent of the lesions (up to 7 mm), i.e. the width of the neoplastic changes. A high correlation has been found between the depth and the width of invasion. Takeshima et al [15] studied 402 microscopic cervical cancers with an invasion of 5 mm or less in depth, and found that an excess of 7 mm horizontal spread was 6.3% in cases with 3 mm invasion, compared to 61% for those with a depth of invasion of 3-5 mm.

Additional pathological parameters include LVS involvement, invasive growth pattern and tumour volume. Confluent growth has been correlated with depth of invasion and width (< 7 mm versus > 7.1 mm) [15]. However, the differentiation between growth patterns such as "fingerlike" and "confluent" is too subjective, making their significance questionable. Oedematous stromal reaction with lymphatic infiltration is not uncommon. The diagnosis of LVSI is not easy and requires the proper identification of an endothelial lining space containing atypical cells. Tissue shrinkage may be misleadingly diagnosed as LVSI. A high correlation between depth of invasion and presence of LVSI has been found. In tumours invading by less than 1 mm, LVSI is very rare (0-8%).

There is no accepted definition for micro-invasive adenocarcinoma. This entity, however, exists. The histological features of early invasive adenocarcinoma include an irregularly infiltrating gland lacking the characteristic pattern of the adenocarcinoma in situ.

Management

Cancer management is tailored to the risk of recurrence, and this is also true for micro-invasive cervical carcinoma. The treatment of micro-invasive cervical carcinoma is confusing, ranging from local excision to radical hysterectomy and pelvic lymphadenectomy, the latter much favoured in the 1960s and 1970s. During the last 20 years, however, there has been a trend towards conservative management. Minimally invasive surgery in low-risk patients is generally carried out in a standard way, while the treatment of women with increased risk should be managed case by case. The major determinants include lesion characteristics, age, patient's desire for further childbearing, menopausal status, history of cancer susceptibility, presence or absence of other pathologies and cancer phobia.

■ Treatment options

Conisation (loop, cold-knife, laser)

The high correlation between tumour-free conisation margins and lack of residual lesions in the upper cervix and uterine corpus suggests that in micro-invasive cervical carcinoma, conisation can replace simple hysterectomy without compromising patient care. Indeed, many studies have demonstrated excellent results. There is no convincing evidence that simple hysterectomy is superior to adequate cone biopsy. Nevertheless, residual disease may occur in the histological specimen. The major advantages of conisation are: 1) it is an outpatient procedure; 2) associated morbidity is minimal; 3) preservation of further childbearing is possible.

Surgical margins are of great importance; unless they are free of disease, it is impossible to assess the true extent of the disease with the risk of not diagnosing occult stage IB tumours. Whether this has any clinical impact is not yet certain. Burghardt et al [3] reported 16 patients with small stage IB (upgraded from stage IA tumours) treated with conisation or simple hysterectomy. None recurred within 5 years. The data, however, are insufficient for drawing useful conclusions. In contrast to CIN, the regression rate of early invasive cervical lesions has not been addressed by many authors in the literature for the obvious reason of an immediate second surgical excision if the margin, particularly the endocervical or deep margin, is positive. The external margin can easily be assessed by colposcopy and cytology for the presence of any residual disease following wound healing. A suspected remaining tumour requires re-conisation. The limited data suggest that some patients with positive cone margins did not have any residual disease in the re-conisation or hysterectomy specimen, and some of those not treated with repeat surgery did not relapse; the majority, however, had recurrence. The role of cytology and colposcopy in the follow-up of these women has not been established, and it is unlikely that sufficient data can be collected. Currently, there is a general consensus that in the presence of positive margins, more common in postmenopausal women, a re-conisation is indicated, which is usually carried out 4 to 6 weeks after the first surgical intervention.

Adequate analysis of the cone specimen by the pathologist is a prerequisite for correct histological staging. Unless the cone is properly handled and studied under the microscope, it cannot be certain that conisation as a definitive treatment is reliable. Residual disease in the post-conisation hysterectomy specimens, in the presence of lesion-free cone margins, may be explained by improper evaluation of the conisation specimen.

Loop excision has gained wide acceptance and is apparently replacing laser and cold-knife conisation [6]. It is a simple technique, as efficient as other cone biopsy methods in removing the entire area of CIN. It also seems to be comparable with cold-knife conisation in diagnosing and treating microcarcinoma of the uterine cervix, provided that a single slice technique is used. If multiple applications of loop conisation are inevitable, cold-knife cone biopsy is the preferred method [16]. Skill and experience are mandatory. Difficulties in completely visualising the cervix, due to atrophy, stenosis or anatomical alterations, require general anaesthesia for performing correct cone biopsies. Anaesthesia is more often needed for re-conisation.

Traditionally, routine post-conisation endocervical curettage is proposed. This is helpful in ruling out invasive lesions high in the cervical canal. The yield is low. If the tissue samples obtained by endocervical curettage contain cancer cells, the disease should not be graded as micro-invasive carcinoma.

Simple hysterectomy

Vaginal and abdominal hysterectomy are equally effective in controlling primary disease. In the stage 1A1 disease, some investigators have suggested an extrafascial hysterectomy for post-menopausal women, and perhaps for those premenopausal patients who have completed childbearing, but there is a significant trend towards more conservative surgical treatment, even in these settings. Simple hysterectomy has also been recommended for treating stage IA1 lesions with LVSI [13]; however, there is no strong evidence to support this view. It has been suggested that patients with stage IA2 tumours require a vaginal or abdominal hysterectomy after cone biopsy, if subsequent fertility is not a consideration. This concept is based on the findings that residual lesions may be present in the remaining cervix, despite negative conisation margins. This risk, however, is very low, provided the cone specimen is adequately studied histologically. Again, there is no consensus on this.

The rate of residual disease in micro-adenocarcinoma is not yet clear; it is perhaps more substantial and warrants a hysterectomy in patients who do not wish to maintain their reproductive capacity.

If the surgical margins are positive, some authors favour performing a hysterectomy immediately for evaluation of the entire lesion, instead of a re-conisation. This approach is inappropriate because if a more advanced invasive tumour is found in the hysterectomy specimen, additional treatment, either lymphadenectomy with or without radical parametrectomy or pelvic irradiation, will be needed. The major disadvantages of this are: 1) a second surgical intervention; 2) the technical difficulties and greater morbidity of radical parametrectomy, compared to radical hysterectomy; 3) pelvic irradiation that could have been avoided. Should a hysterectomy be indicated, the cone biopsy can be repeated and sent for rapid examination. In the absence of more advanced disease in frozen sections, a hysterectomy can safely be completed.

Radical hysterectomy

A modified radical hysterectomy is mostly recommended, and a classic type III radical hysterectomy is rarely performed routinely [7]. Sevin et al [13] suggested a modified radical hysterectomy as an alternative to simple hysterectomy for patients with stage IA2 disease. Even if the specific disease survival rate after modified radical hysterectomy is excellent (100%), it appears to be an overtreatment in almost all cases. The incidence of parametrial involvement is extremely rare - perhaps 0%. Indeed, more and more authors assume that conisation or a simple hysterectomy is just as efficient as radical hysterectomy, with considerably less morbidity [14].

Lymphadenectomy

Evaluation of the pelvic lymph nodes in stage IA2 lesions by lymphadenectomy (retroperitoneal or laparoscopic) has been carried out [2] based on an approximate 2% incidence of microscopic nodal involvement [4]. Recent reports, however, have demonstrated slightly higher incidence rates of 3% to 5%. In spite of this, whether lymphadectomy is justified in all cases has yet to be determined. Imaging techniques are not useful in disclosing microscopic lymph node metastases. The therapeutic value of lymph node dissection in the presence of positive nodes has been reported in most studies to be approximately 50%, i.e. only every second patient benefits from lymphadenectomy. Thus, the therapeutic benefit of pelvic lymphadenectomy in stage IA2 tumours is very small and would apply to only one or two out of 100 patients. One concern of lymphadenectomy, in addition to its invasive nature and associated morbidity, is its resulting host defence impairment in early stages as suggested by accumulating evidence [11].

Radical vaginal trachelectomy

This is a novel, fertility sparing procedure which is valuable in well-selected patients with early-stage cervical carcinoma [5]. Successful pregnancies are definitely possible after this operation [10]. During surgery, the uterine cervix is amputated 1 cm below the isthmus, and an adequate amount of parametrium is removed. The uterine corpus is preserved. The procedure is combined with laparoscopic pelvic lymphadenectomy. There is a paucity of data concerning the precise indication for this surgical technique. It is apparently indicated in high-risk, young patients with early stage disease for whom childbearing is of concern and when there is a risk of parametrial involvement.

Radiation therapy

The author's experience (unpublished data) is in accordance with others, suggesting that microscopic cervical lesions can be effectively treated with intracavity high or low dose rate brachytherapy without external beam irradiation [8, 12]. The place of radiation therapy, however, is controversial and it is rarely used. The recommended radiation dose is 60-75 Gy to point A.

■ General considerations

In planning therapy, the following issues should be taken into consideration:

1) As with all stages, micro-carcinoma of the uterine cervix is a disease continuum, and therefore, the actual depth and width of the neoplastic changes, i.e. the extent/volume of the tumour, have an important prognostic/predictive value;

2) extra-uterine spread is almost always microscopic, and since any diagnostic tool other than histology cannot detect microscopic involvement, other prognostic parameters reflecting the biological behaviour of the tumour are perhaps predictive in microscopic spread and are also important.

3) The fate of microscopic lymph node (parametrial) metastases is unknown, and the role of the lymph nodes in the host defence has recently been appreciated.

4) In stage IA1 disease, the incidence of pelvic lymph node metastases is < 1%, and the involvement of the cardinal ligament is unlikely. The role of LVSI in predicting the presence of extra-uterine spread is still controversial, although there are data suggesting possible significance. The actual depth of invasion can have predictive power; lesions with < 1 mm in depth have minimal or no risk of metastasising. The extent of horizontal spread (increased tumour volume) is apparently of predictive value. There is no evidence that other prognostic markers, including molecular factors, can be routinely used in predicting microscopic metastasis.

5) In stage IA2 lesions, the incidence of pelvic node involvement is approximately 2 to 5%, with negligible risk of parametrial involvement. As with stage IA1 disease, further studies are warranted to determine the predictive value of LVSI, the width of neoplastic changes and other particular molecular markers.

6) Does a 2% to 5% risk of incidence justify 95% to 98% unnecessary major surgery?

7) Although the prognosis of recurrent disease is poor, some local recurrence can be salvaged.

8) There is no convincing evidence that hysterectomy is superior to correct cone biopsy in eradicating the primary squamous cervical lesion, although it may be in the presence of micro-adenocarcinoma or other unfavourable histological types.

9) The different forms of hysterectomy, including abdominal, vaginal, laparoscopic or laparoscopically-assisted vaginal hysterectomy, have no impact on outcome.

10) Simple hysterectomy is of no use in controlling extra-uterine spread.

11) Simple hysterectomy combined with pelvic lymphadenectomy does not include the parametrium (the conduit for cancer cells towards the pelvic nodes).

12) Modified radical hysterectomy does not remove the lateral parametrium.

13) Whether or not the lateral parametrium should be excised during radical vaginal trachelectomy remains to be determined.

14) The more radical the surgery, the higher the risk of associated morbidity.

15) Oophorectomy or salpingo-oophorectomy do not influence outcome.

Recommended strategies *(fig 1)*

Stage IA1 squamous cell lesions

The management of stage IA1 squamous cell carcinoma has generally been agreed upon. Most patients are treated conservatively, either by cone biopsy or simple hysterectomy. There is no evidence that hysterectomy is superior to conisation. For young patients who wish to preserve their childbearing function, adequate cone biopsy is the treatment of choice. In the author's view, additional indications, including fear of cancer, patient wishes, menopausal status and improper histological evaluation of the cone specimen, are needed to perform a hysterectomy. All kinds of hysterectomy are equally effective. There is no need to remove normal looking ovaries unless indicated. The risk of lymph node involvement is too small to substantiate lymph node dissection. Since parametrial involvement is perhaps 0%, there is no place for modified radical hysterectomy or radical vaginal trachelectomy.

Stage IA1   Stage IA2

Therapeutic conisation   Therapeutic conisation
Hysterectomy*   Pelvic lymphadenectomy
                                                               Hysterectomy*

Surgical margins
                                                               Surgical margins

                   Involved

                                                                              Involved

Clear ◄——— Reconisation
                                                   Clear ◄——— Reconisation

Follow-up
                                                   Pelvic nodes (?)

                                          Negative   Positive

                                          Follow-up   Modified radical hysterectomy
                                                               Radical vaginal trachelectomy

                                                               Follow-up

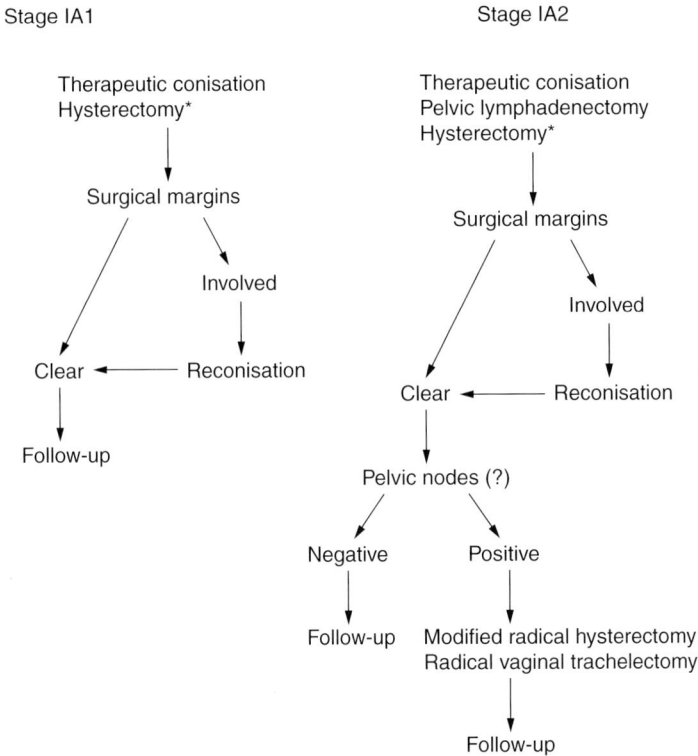

Figure 1. *A general algorithm for treating micro-invasive carcinoma of the uterine cervix. The treatment, however, can be individualised based on risk factors. (Hysterectomy* = only in the presence of additional indication.)*

Stage IA2 squamous cell lesions

Management of stage IA2 squamous cell lesions continues to be debated. The data currently available are insufficient to allow the gynaecological oncology community to give firm guidelines regarding the appropriate treatment for patients with stage IA2 cervical carcinoma. For local control, conisation or simple hysterectomy, the latter, mostly in the presence of additional indications (including postmenopausal age), is adequate. There is no convincing evidence for the use of modified or extended radical hysterectomy. In spite of this, a modified radical hysterectomy has been recommended and is used in many centres world-wide. The risk of parametrial involvement is increased in the presence of lymph node metastasis, particularly when more than one node is involved, and there may be a place for modified radical hysterectomy in such cases. Radical vaginal trachelectomy is a valid alternative to radical hysterectomy if childbearing is to be preserved. Pelvic lymphadenectomy is recommended, but is not substantiated as a standard procedure, and perhaps should be tailored according to risk factors.

In the presence of involved cone margins, irrespective of stage IA1 or IA2, re-conisation is mandatory prior to any additional treatment to rule out invasive cancer that may be present in the upper part of the cervix.

For micro-adenocarcinoma, a simple hysterectomy is recommended after adequate conisation, because of the increased incidence of residual disease. However, special consideration is needed in women who wish to maintain their reproductive capacity. They should be informed that there is no guarantee of the absence of residual disease that may be invasive carcinoma, and that they are at risk of recurrence [1].

Follow-up

Close follow-up is particularly important for patients treated with conisation. Follow-up visits are required every three months for two years, every 6 months for the following two years and yearly afterwards. In addition to routine examination, colposcopy and cytology are mandatory on each occasion. Any abnormality should be evaluated without delay. Post-treatment surveillance is not less important after hysterectomy. Imaging techniques, especially vaginal ultrasonography, are helpful in follow-up; their place however, has not been determined. The same is true for serum markers such as SCC.

After cone biopsy treatment of micro-adenocarcinoma, aggressive endocervical cytology every 3 months for three years and every six months for an undetermined number of additional years is highly recommended.

Future avenues

In the author's view, the treatment of even micro-invasive cervical carcinoma should be individualised. This is based on molecular biological factors, particularly on molecular genetic changes. Cancer is a heterogeneous disease from the very beginning, requiring tailored treatment. This is more relevant because micro-invasive lesions represent a disease continuum, and any compartmentalisation, i.e. stage, is artificial and does not represent homogeneous tumours.

References

[1] Azodi M, Chambers SK, Rutherford TJ, Kohorn EI, Schwartz P, Chambers JT. Adenocarcinoma in situ of the cervix: management and outcome. *Gynecol Oncol* 1999 ; 73 : 348-353

[2] Buckely SL, Tritz DM, Van Le L, Higgins R, Sevin BU, Ueland FR et al. Lymph node metastasis and prognosis in patients with stage IA2 cervical cancer. *Gynecol Oncol* 1996 ; 63 : 4-9

[3] Burghardt E, Girardi F, Lahousen M, Pickel H, Tamussino K. Microinvasive carcinoma of the uterine cervix (International Federation of Gynecology and Obstetrics Stage IA). *Cancer* 1991 ; 67 : 1037-1045

[4] Creasman WT. Stage IA cancer of the cervix: finally some resolution of definition and treatment? *Gynecol Oncol* 1999 ; 74 : 163-164

[5] Dargent D, Brun JL, Roy M, Mathevet P, Remy ILA. Trachélectomie élargie une alternative à l'hystérectomie radicale dans le traitement des cancers infiltrants développés sur la face externe du col utérin. *J Obstét Gynécol* 1994 ; 2 : 285-292

[6] Kennedy AW, Belinson JL, Wirth S, Taylor J. The role of loop electric excision procedure in the diagnosis and management of early invasive cervical cancer. *Int J Gynecol Cancer* 1995 ; 5 : 117-125

[7] Magrina JF, Goodrich MA, Lidner TK, Weaver AL, Cornella JL, Podratz KC. Modified radical hysterectomy in the treatment of early squamous cervical cancer. *Gynecol Oncol* 1999 ; 72 : 183-186

[8] Nelson JH, Averette HE, Richart RM. Detection, diagnostic evaluation and treatment of dysplasia and early carcinoma of the cervix. *CA Cancer J Clin* 1975 ; 25 : 134-141

[9] Östör AG. Pandora's box or Ariadne's thread. Definition and prognostic significance of microinvasion in the uterne cervix squamous lesion. *Pathol Annu* 1995 ; 30 : 103-136

[10] Roy M, Plante M. Pregnancies after radical vaginal trachelectomy for early-stage cervical cancer. *Am J Obstet Gynecol* 1998 ; 179 : 1491-1506

[11] Santin AD, Parham GP. Routine lymph node dissection in the treatment of early stage cancer: are we doing the right thing? *Gynecol Oncol* 1998 ; 68 : 1-3

[12] Seski JC, Abell MR, Morley GW. Microinvasive squamous carcinoma of the cervix: definition, histology analysis, late results of treatment. *Obstet Gynecol* 1977 ; 50 : 410-418

[13] Sevin BU, Nadji M, Averette HE, Hilsenbeck S, Smith D, Lampe B. Microinvasive carcinoma of the cervix. *Cancer* 1992 ; 70 : 2121-2128

[14] Shingleton HM. Surgery for cervical cancer a time for reassessment. *Gynecol Oncol* 1998 ; 69 : 8-13

[15] Takeshima N, Yanoh T, Nagai K, Hirai Y, Hasumi K. Assessment of the revised International Federation of Gynecology and Obstetrics staging for early invasive squamous cell carcinoma. *Gynecol Oncol* 1999 ; 74 : 165-169

[16] Tseng CJ, Liang CC, Lin CT, Huang KG, Chou HH, Chang TC et al. A study of diagnostic failure of loop conisation in microinvasive carcinoma of the cervix. *Gynecol Oncol* 1999 ; 73 : 91-95

Chapter 7

Radical abdominal hysterectomy for stage I and II cervical carcinoma

Raimund Winter, Karl Tamussino

R Winter, M.D., Full Professor.
K Tamussino, M.D.
Department of Obstetrics and Gynecology, University of Graz, Auenbruggerplatz, 14, A-8036 Graz, Austria.

Radical abdominal hysterectomy for stage I and II cervical carcinoma

R Winter, K Tamussino

Abstract. — *The advantages of surgical treatment of stage IB to IIB cervical cancer include the precise determination of the spread of the tumour and the preservation of ovarian function and sexual function, particularly in younger patients. Radical abdominal hysterectomy as described by Wertheim entails resection of the parametrial tissue and a vaginal cuff as indicated. Systematic pelvic lymphadenectomy is performed before radical hysterectomy. Sytematic lymphadenectomy removes more lymph nodes than sampling lymphadenectomy. Intraoperative frozen section histology of the lymph nodes helps plan the rest of the operation. The lymph node status and the tumour size (volume) are the most important prognostic factors in patients with surgically treated cervical cancer. The risk of parametrial and para-aortic metastases is high in patients with positive pelvic lymph nodes. In these patients the parametrium is resected at the pelvic wall as described by Latzko and the lymphadenectomy is extended to the para-aortic region. The length of the resected vaginal cuff depends on the size of the tumour and on whether it extends to the vagina. The margin of healthy tissue should be 2 to 3 cm. Radical parametrectomy is an option for younger patients in whom an invasive cervical cancer is found incidentally in a uterus removed at simple hysterectomy. Lower urinary tract dysfunction (micturition disorders, stress incontinence, impaired sensation) is the most common complication after radical hysterectomy, occurring in 20% to 80% of patients. Ureterovaginal or vesicovaginal fistulas occur in 2% and 0.9%, respectively. Urinary tract infection occurs in 5% to 10% of postoperative patients. Depending on the definition, the rate of febrile morbidity is 25% to 50%. Lymphocysts occur in up to 20% of patients, even if the pelvic peritoneum is left open. Most lymphocysts are asymptomatic and detected only at imaging studies such as computed tomography during follow-up. Surgical mortality is less than 1%.*

Five-year survival rates depend on tumour size and on the status of the lymph nodes. The survival rate of patients with small tumours (<2.5 cm³) is 91%, regardless of node status, whereas that of patients with large tumours (10 - 50 cm³) is 70%. Overall, the five-year survival rate of patients with stage IB disease is 91% for patients with negative nodes and 66% for those with positive nodes. The survival rate of patients with stage IIB disease with negative nodes is 77% as opposed to 46% for those with positive nodes. Survival is also associated with the number of involved lymph nodes and lymph node groups and the size of the metastases. The survival rate of patients with one positive lymph node is 70%, compared with 37% for those with four or more positive nodes. The survival rate of patients with microscopic metastases in the lymph nodes is 68%, compared to less than 40% for those with gross, bulky nodes.

Keywords: cervical cancer, radical hysterectomy, surgical treatment.

Introduction

Surgery is used to treat a spectrum of invasive cervical cancers of different sizes and histologies. A detailed appreciation of the spread of cervical cancer is a prerequisite for surgical cure. The advantages of surgical therapy compared with radiotherapy include the precise staging of the extent of the disease and the preservation of ovarian function [7, 8]. Sexual function is less impaired after surgery than after radiotherapy, particularly in younger patients. Progress in anaesthesia and postoperative care mean that most older patients tolerate radical hysterectomy as well as younger patients [19]. The indication for surgical treatment of cervical cancer is influenced by the age and medical status of the patient, by the clinical stage of the disease, and by the training and personal experience of the gynaecologic oncologist [21].

Surgical radicality

The term radical (or extended) hysterectomy denotes extirpation of the uterus with a vaginal cuff and the attendant tissue of the parametrium and paracolpos [7, 8, 33]. Pelvic lymphadenectomy [35] is also a part of the operation. Removal of the tubes and ovaries, discussed below, is not a component of radical hysterectomy. Discussions of surgical radicality centre on how much of the parametrial tissue and the upper vagina are resected, i.e. on how much clearance from the tumour is necessary.

The extent of surgical radicality depends on the size of the tumour and whether there are signs of spread to the parametrial tissue or vagina. The parametrial tissue lateral to the uterus is the structure through which the disease spreads to the pelvic wall [6]. Parametrial involvement usually comprises discontinuous spread to lymphatic vessels and lymph nodes in the parametrium. Continuous extension to the parametrial tissue is less common. The frequency of parametrial involvement is associated with the size (volume) of the tumour [6, 8]. The topographic localisation of metastases in the parametrial tissue is unpredictable. Positive parametrial nodes can be found close to the cervix, near the pelvic sidewall, or in between [13]. Thus, partial resection of the lateral parametrial tissue may entail a risk of leaving involved parametrial lymph nodes in situ and is appropriate only for small tumours with negative pelvic nodes at intraoperative frozen section analysis.

The radical hysterectomy originally described by Wertheim [34] entails division of the parametrium halfway between the cervix and the pelvic sidewall. Wertheim's pupil Latzko [18] extended the resection of the parametrium laterally to the pelvic wall. TeLinde described a modified radical hysterectomy which entails resection of the bit of parametrium between the cervix and the ureter and a small vaginal cuff [25]. It is not clear if this operation offers a better chance for cure than simple hysterectomy without resection of parametrial tissue or a vaginal cuff. In 1974 Piver et al [25] attempted to classify the various modifications of radical hysterectomy.

The vesicocervical and vesicouterine tissue anteriorly and the sacrouterine ligament posteriorly are rarely involved in the spread of cervical cancer. The length of the anterior tissue is limited by the proximity of the bladder to the cervix so that extended resection is not an issue. The sacrouterine ligament, which does not contain lymph nodes, can be resected posteriorly at the rectum. The length of the vaginal cuff depends on the size and extension of the tumour. The margin should be 2-3 cm from the tumour. If the upper third of the vagina is resected, the sagittal vesicovaginal ligament is resected as well [1].

The extended hysterectomies originally described by Wertheim [34] and Latzko [18] have been repeatedly modified with the aims of tailoring the operation to the size of the tumour and reducing the rate of postoperative complications. Results of these modifications are available only in retrospective series.

■ Salpingo-oophorectomy

As mentioned above, removal of the tubes and ovaries is not part of radical hysterectomy per se. The incidence of ovarian metastasis in clinical stage I squamous cell carcinoma of the cervix is less than 0.5% [1]. Thus routine salpingo-oophorectomy in premenopausal women is not indicated. If in a young woman adjuvant radiotherapy is a possibility, the ovaries should be transposed high into the respective paracolic gutters out of the pelvis [9, 22]. This is done by mobilising the respective infundibulopelvic ligament cranially. On the left side the infundibulopelvic ligament should remain under the descending colon. Marking with a haemostatic clip will help the radiation oncologist to identify the ovaries. If chemotherapy is planned the ovaries can be left in the pelvis.

Surgical anatomy

■ Potential spaces in the pelvis

The potential spaces in the pelvis shown in figure 1 were first described by Peham and Amreich [23]. These spaces are essential to define the surgical anatomy for radical hysterectomy. The spaces are the bilateral paravesical and pararectal spaces and the median prevesical, vesicovaginal and vesicocervical, rectovaginal, and retrorectal spaces (*fig 1*). The prevesical space (space of Retzius) and the retrorectal space are not important for radical hysterectomy.

The paravesical space becomes accessible after dividing the round ligament. The anatomic landmark is the obliterated umbilical artery with the vesicoumbilical fascia beneath it. These structures mark the medial border of the paravesical space, which curves anteriorly along the back of the symphysis. The anterior border is the posterior aspect of the symphysis, the lateral border is the fascia overlying the internal obturator muscle, the inferior border is the pubic portion of the levator ani muscle, and the posterior border is the anterior aspect of the parametrium and paracolpium (cardinal ligament). For radical hysterectomy, traction is put on the obliterated umbilical artery and the space is developed with blunt dissection in the areolar tissue down to the pelvic floor.

The pararectal space curves anteriorly in front of the sacrum. It is limited anteriorly by the posterior aspect of the parametrium (cardinal ligament), medially by the rectal pillar and the fascia overlying the rectum, laterally by the internal iliac artery and vein, and posteriorly by the anterior aspect of the sacrum. The space is developed with blunt dissection curving anteriorly after identifying the ureter medially and the internal iliac vessels laterally.

The vesicocervical and vesicovaginal spaces are accessed after dividing the peritoneum of the vesicouterine fold. This space is limited anteriorly by the posterior aspect of the bladder, posteriorly by the anterior aspect of the cervix and vagina, and laterally by the vesicocervical and vesicovaginal ligament (bladder pillar). Caudally the space obliterates at the level of the internal urethral orifice.

The rectovaginal space is opened by incising the peritoneum in the pouch of Douglas (posterior cul-de-sac) and bluntly developing the plane between the rectum and vagina

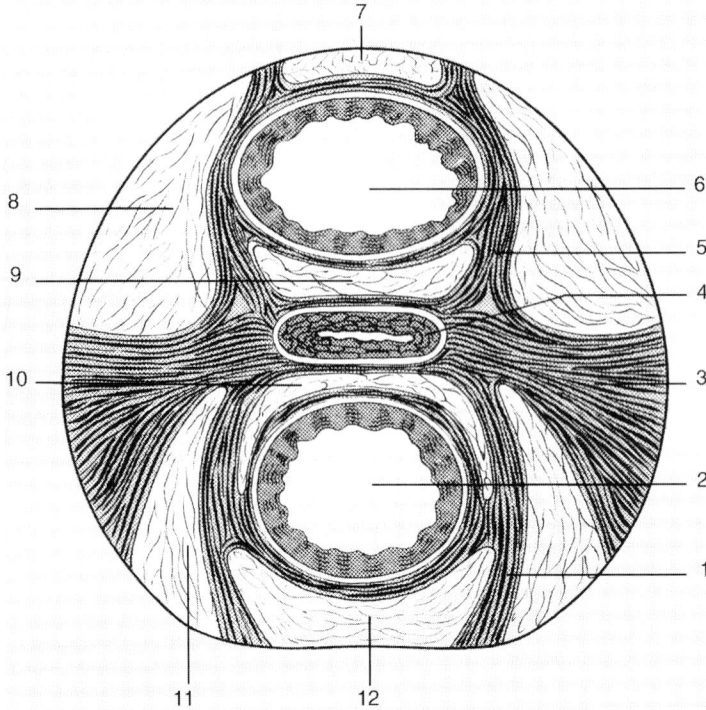

Figure 1. *Schematic representation of the potential spaces and connective tissue structures in the pelvis according to von Peham and Amreich* [23].
1. Bladder; 2. bladder pillar (vesicouterine ligament); 3. vagina; 4. cardinal ligament; 5. rectum; 6. rectal pillar (uterosacral ligament); 7. prevesical space (retropubic space, space of Retzius); 8. paravesical space; 9. vesico-vaginal space; 10. rectovaginal space; 11. pararectal space; 12. retrorectal space.
(From Burghardt E, Webb MJ, Monaghan JM, Kindermann G. Surgical Gynecologic Oncology. © Georg Thieme Verlag, 1993, with permission.)

along the pelvic curve. The space is limited anteriorly by the posterior wall of the vagina, posteriorly by the anterior wall of the rectum, and laterally by the sacrouterine ligaments and rectal pillars.

The parametria are condensations of the connective tissue of the endopelvic fascia [33]. They are the scaffolding for the blood and lymphatic vessels and nerves supplying the pelvic organs. The most important part of the endopelvic fascia is the cardinal ligament. It begins below the uterine artery and is continuous with the paracolpos inferiorly. The cardinal ligament is in the frontal plane intitially and then follows the curvature of the pelvis to become almost horizontal. It lies between the cervix and the pelvic sidewall and separates the paravesical space from the pararectal space. The anterior part of the parametrium consists of the superficial part of the vesicocervical ligament, which lies above the ureter, and of the deep part of the vesicovaginal ligament, which runs sagitally with the bladder pillar. The vesicocervical ligament has to be divided to mobilise the ureter. Depending on the size of the vaginal cuff to be resected, the vesicovaginal ligament has to be resected in part or in its entirety.

The posterior condensation of the endopelvic fascia (the sacrouterine ligament and the rectal pillar) extends from the posterior aspect of the cervix to the sacrum. It consists of the superficial part of the sacrouterine ligament and of the deep part of the rectal pillar. Laterally it lies against the posterior aspect of the lateral parametrium; development of the pararectal space transforms it into a sagittal structure.

■ Vessels and nerves

The parametrial tissue is the scaffolding for blood vessels and nerves to and from the pelvic organs. While the surgically relevant veins run straight across the lateral parametrium, the autonomous nerves of the sympathetic and parasympathetic plexus run to their respective organs sagitally in the rectal and bladder pillars. The bladder and rectal pillars can be thought of as crossing the lateral parametrium (cardinal ligament) at a right angle.

Lymphadenectomy

Careful removal of the primary tumour and the lymphatic system draining it is a fundamental principle of surgical oncology. Pelvic lymphadenectomy is performed before radical hysterectomy per se, and sets up the latter operation [7, 35]. The pelvic nodes are submitted for frozen section histology as they are removed and their status influences the radicality of the hysterectomy. The probability of parametrial and para-aortic lymph node involvement increases with the number of positive pelvic nodes.

The lymph node bearing tissue is exposed by dividing the infundibulopelvic or the ovarian ligament. A systematic lymphadenectomy requires incising the adventitial tissue surrounding the major vessels and then removing the entire lymphatic fatty tissue around and between the major vessels. Pelvic lymphadenectomy is performed from the femoral ring up to the bifurcation of the aorta. The surgical field in the obturator fossa extends from the inferior margin of the external iliac vein down to the pelvic floor. The obturator artery and vein are clipped and resected, taking care to spare the nerve *(fig 2)*. Then the iliac vessels are mobilised from the pelvic wall to remove the lymphatic fatty tissue lateral to and between the major vessels. This exposes the lumbosacral plexus lateral to the common iliac vessels. In contrast, a staging lymphadenectomy removes only the nodes ventral to the external iliac and distal half of the common iliac vessels and the obturator nodes above the obturator nerve.

The surgical field for para-aortic lymphadenectomy [35] extends from the bifurcation of the aorta to the upper margin of the left renal vein. The lateral border of the surgical field is marked by the ureter. There are a number of approaches to the paraaortic region. A direct approach is gained by extending cranially the incision of the pelvic peritoneum along the aorta to the duodenojejunal flexure. The upper margin of the left renal vein is exposed by bluntly mobilising upward the horizontal part of the duodenum. The second approach involves dividing the peritoneum in the right paracolic gutter up to the right colic flexure. The colon can be mobilised medially to completely expose the para-aortic field. The para-aortic region can also be exposed by dividing the peritoneum in the left paracolic gutter up to the left colonic flexure and reflecting the descending colon medially.

After exposure is obtained the right ovarian vein is ligated and divided at its origin from the vena cava. The inferior mesenteric artery is exposed. This artery is preserved but can be sacrificied because there are anastomoses with the superior mesenteric artery. Systematic paraaortic lymphadenectomy entails complete removal of the lymphatic fatty tissue around the aorta and vena cava. By rolling the vessels to one side

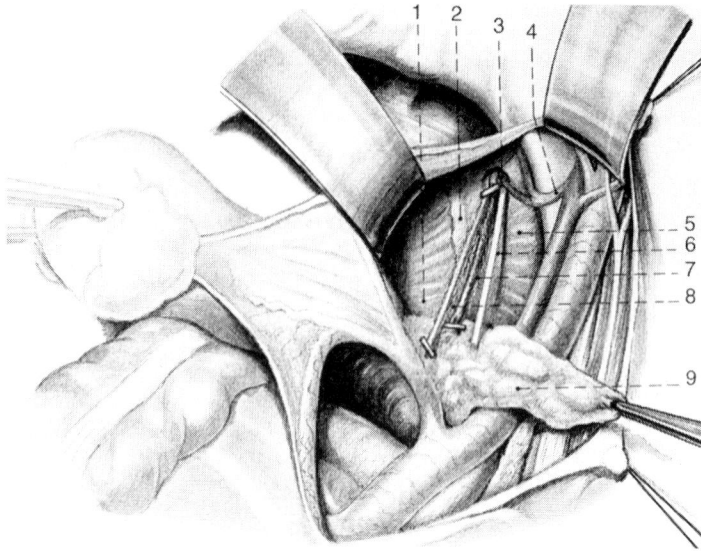

Figure 2. *Lymphadenectomy in the obturator fossa. The lymphatic channels have been divided at the lymphatic lacuna and the obtutrator vessels have been clipped before resection. The lymphatic tissue is dissected in a cephalad direction, taking care to preserve the obturator nerve. The tissue is removed en bloc after dividing the obturator vessels. The lateral pelvic wall, the arcus tendineus, and the pelvic floor are exposed.*
1. Iliac portion of the levator ani muscle; 2. arcus tendineus fasciae pelvis; 3. obturator fossa; 4. accessory obturator vein; 5. internal obturator muscle; 6. obturator nerve; 7. obturator vein; 8. obturator artery; 9. lymphatic tissue in the obturator fossa.
(From Burghardt E, Webb MJ, Monaghan JM, Kindermann G. Surgical Gynecologic Oncology. © Georg Thieme Verlag, 1993, with permission.)

and then the other, it is usually possible to clear the area behind the vessels without ligating the lumbar vessels [35]. The sympathetic plexus on both sides is preserved. The anatomy of the vessels in the para-aortic region varies. Accessory arteries are encountered more often than accessory veins. While veins can be ligated without consequence, accessory arteries to the kidneys are end arteries and should not be divided.

There is usually a large lymph node on the anterior aspect of the lower vena cava to the right of the aortic bifurcation. A venous tributary from this node empties directly into the vena cava and should be clipped before removing the node.

Para-aortic lymphadenectomy is completed by resecting the left infundibulopelvic ligament. The left ovarian vein is ligated at its origin from the left renal vein. The ligament is dissected from the posterior aspect of the descending mesocolon. Branches to the mesenterium and the ureter are ligated or cauterised and divided.

Radical abdominal hysterectomy

The extent of the resection of the parametrium (cardinal ligament) laterally and an appropriate vaginal cuff are important. The issue of salpingo-oophorectomy is discussed above. Pelvic lymphadenectomy is performed before the radical hysterectomy and exposes the parametrium and paracolpos.

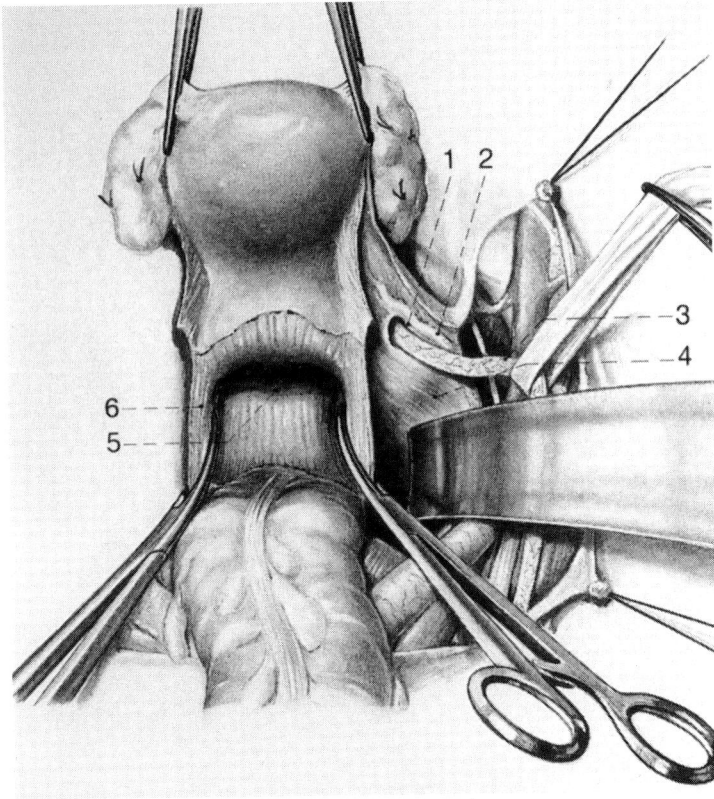

Figure 3. *Clamping of the uterosacral ligaments (rectal pillars). The uterus is pulled anteriorly toward the symphysis and a retractor is in the right pararectal space. The ureter has been completely freed from the peritoneum down to where it enters its canal in the cardinal ligament; it is retracted with a vessel loop. The peritoneum has been incised down to the rectal pillar and in the cul-de-sac. The rectum has been freed from the vagina and from the medial aspects of the uterosacral ligaments.*
1. Ureteral canal; 2. uterine artery; 3. ureter; 4. posterior aspect of the cardinal ligament; 5. rectovaginal space; 6. rectal pillar.
(From Burghardt E, Webb MJ, Monaghan JM, Kindermann G. Surgical Gynecologic Oncology. © Georg Thieme Verlag, 1993, with permission.)

A midline incision is made and can be extended above the umbilicus as required. The contents of the abdominal cavity are systematically inspected and palpated. The retroperitoneal compartment on the right side is opened by dividing the round and infundibulopelvic or ovarian ligaments. The paravesical and pararectal spaces are developed and a systematic lymphadenectomy is performed. The procedure is repeated on the left side and the lymph nodes are sent for frozen section histology. The status of the lymph nodes helps to plan the rest of the operation [7, 35].

Next the ureter is dissected from the peritoneum all the way down to where it enters the parametrium. The peritoneum of the pouch of Douglas is incised and the rectovaginal space is developed. The ventral and lateral aspects of the rectum are exposed to develop the rectal pillar (sacrouterine ligament). The rectal pillars, which lie in a sagittal plane, can be clamped and divided close to the rectum (*fig 3*). A pack is placed in the space.

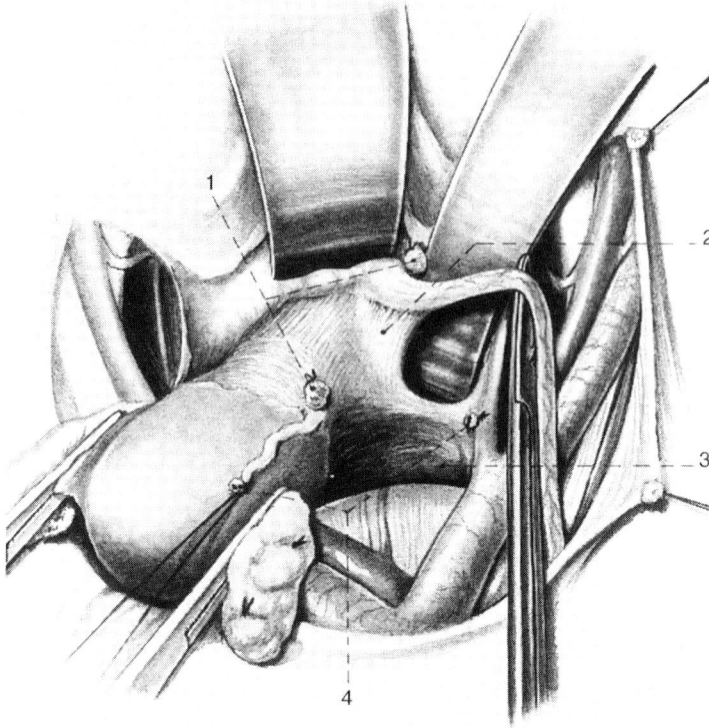

Figure 4. *The right ureter has been dissected out of its canal in the right cardinal ligament and is retracted to expose the vesicocervical and vesicovaginal ligament (bladder pillar). One retractor holds the bladder, the other is in the paravesical space.*
1. Pedicles of the vesicocervical ligament: 2. vesicovaginal ligament; 3. posterior aspect of the cardinal ligament; 4. uterine artery pedicles.
(From Burghardt E, Webb MJ, Monaghan JM, Kindermann G. Surgical Gynecologic Oncology. © Georg Thieme Verlag, 1993, with permission.)

The vesicouterine peritoneum is incised and the vesicocervical and vesicovaginal spaces are developed by dissecting the bladder down off the cervix and upper vagina. The uterine artery is ligated at its origin from the internal iliac artery and is dissected medially toward the uterus. This exposes the roof of the ureteral canal in the cardinal ligament. The ureter is thus freed to where it enters the bladder *(fig 4)*. If a considerable vaginal cuff has to be resected, the deep sagittal bladder pillar (vesicovaginal ligament) is clamped and divided *(fig 5)*.

Now the uterus is freed anteriorly. The lateral parametrium can now be divided halfway between the cervix and the pelvic wall, as described by Wertheim [34]. This extent of parametrial resection seems adequate for tumours less than 2.5 cm in diameter and if the pelvic lymph nodes are negative. Larger tumours and those with positive pelvic nodes require resection of the entire parametrium directly at the pelvic sidewall as described by Latzko [18] *(fig 6)*.

The size of the vaginal cuff depends on the extent of the tumour. The margin of healthy tissue should be 2-3 cm *(fig 7)*. The cut edges of the vagina are oversewn and the vagina is left open for drainage. The pelvic peritoneum is also left open. Two passive drains are brought out through the vagina and are removed after 3-5 days. A suprapubic

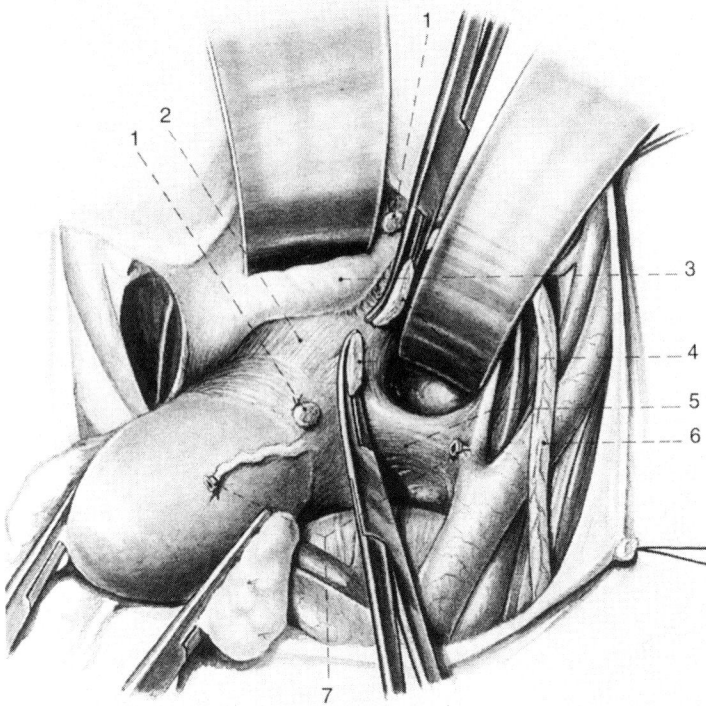

Figure 5. *The bladder pillar (vesicovaginal ligament) is clamped and cut. This step, and the one shown in figure 7, is probably crucial for the degree of postoperative urinary dysfunction. The right cardinal ligament is now completely exposed and can be divided wherever desired.*
1. Pedicles of the vesicocervical ligament; 2. vagina; 3. bladder; 4. cut vesicovaginal ligament; 5. posterior aspect of the cardinal ligament; 6. ureter; 7. uterine artery pedicles.
(From Burghardt E, Webb MJ, Monaghan JM, Kindermann G. Surgical Gynecologic Oncology. © Georg Thieme Verlag, 1993, with permission.)

catheter is inserted. The catheter is removed when residual urine volumes are consistently less than 100 mL or when the patient is comfortable with intermittent self-catheterisation.

Radical parametrectomy after hysterectomy

Radical parametrectomy and excision of the upper vagina are indicated for young women with an incidental finding of invasive cervical carcinoma after conventional hysterectomy [36]. The operation is performed 6-8 weeks after hysterectomy to allow the vaginal vault to heal. The pelvic anatomy is somewhat altered after hysterectomy. The base of the bladder usually lies over the vaginal vault and can obscure the entry into the vesicovaginal space. The anatomy of the parametria is unaffected.

The initial steps of the pelvic lymphadenectomy are the same as at radical hysterectomy. A prosthesis is inserted into the vagina and kept under tension by an assistant. Putting the vagina on traction facilitates the dissection of the ureters and development of the parametria. After division of the bladder and rectal pillars, straight clamps can be put on the angles of the vagina and the prosthesis can be removed. The parametrium and paracolpos can now be resected with an adequate vaginal cuff [36].

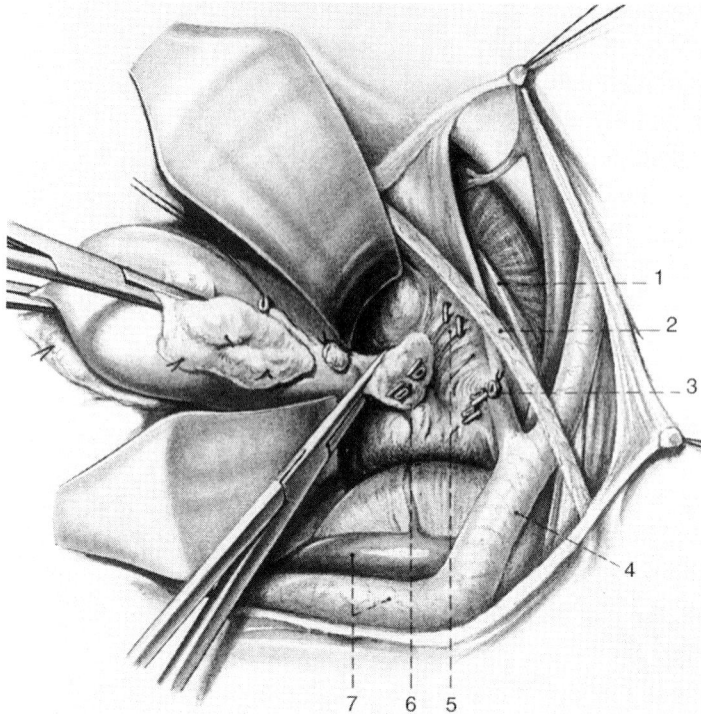

Figure 6. *The right cardinal ligament has been clipped and divided directly at the pelvic wall. The uterus is pulled to the left and a straight clamp is on the middle of the cardinal ligament. The paravesical and pararectal spaces are opened up with retractors.*
1. Obturator nerve; 2. ureter; 3. uterine artery pedicle; 4. common iliac artery; 5. clips where the cardinal ligament has been resected at the pelvic wall; 6. medial pedicle of the cardinal ligament; 7. left common iliac vessels.
(From Burghardt E, Webb MJ, Monaghan JM, Kindermann G. Surgical Gynecologic Oncology. © Georg Thieme Verlag, 1993, with permission.)

Complications of radical hysterectomy

Most complications become apparent while the patient is still in the hospital. The most common problem after radical hysterectomy is lower urinary tract dysfunction, which occurs in 20% to 80% of patients. The most common symptoms are impaired bladder sensation and voiding dysfunction. Bladder function improves over the years, particularly in patients who do not receive radiotherapy [28]. The extent of the resection of the vaginal cuff and division of the vesicovaginal ligament appears to be related to the degree of postoperative urinary tract dysfunction [29]. Stress incontinence can develop in approximately 20% of patients [28] and pre-exisiting stress incontinence can be exacerbated.

Preoperatively patients should be counselled about lower urinary tract dysfunction and the management of suprapubic catheters and intermittent self-catheterisation should be discussed. Postoperatively the patient should be instructed to void every 2-4 hours to avoid overdistension and damage to the detrusor muscle. Urinary tract infection should be ruled out, particularly in patients with residual urine. The rate of postoperative urinary tract infection is about 10%. Prophylactic oral antibiotics do not prevent urinary

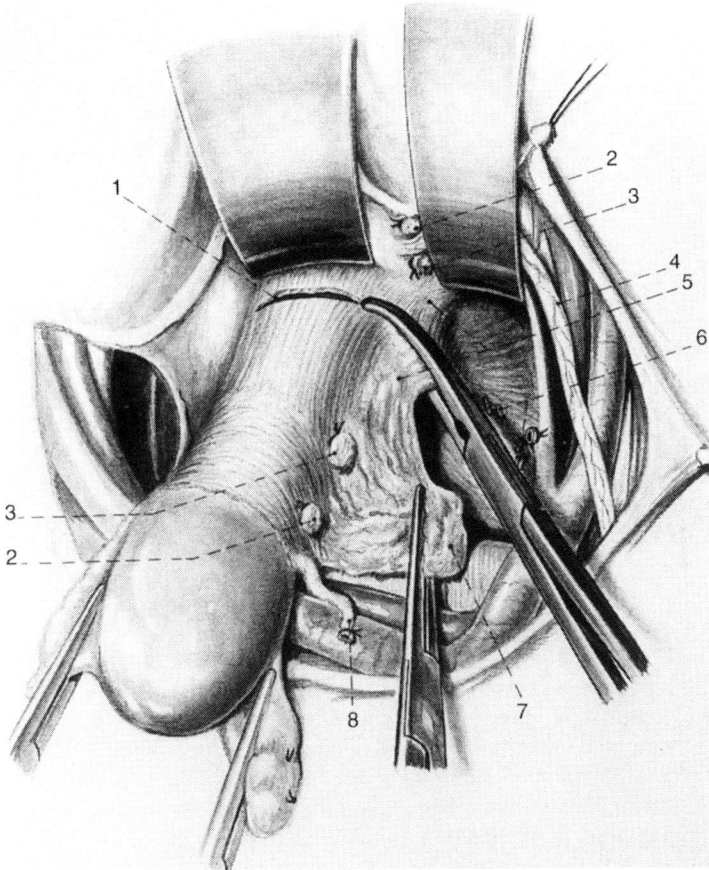

Figure 7. *A Wertheim clamp is placed on the paravaginal tissue at the level where the vagina is to be transected. The uterus is pulled toward the sacrum. One retractor holds back the bladder and a second opens the paravesical space and protects the ureter. This step, and the one shown in figure 5, is probably crucial for the degree of postoperative urinary dysfunction.*
1. Incision of the vagina; 2. pedicles of the vesicocervical ligament; 3. pedicles of the vesicovaginal ligament; 4. ureter; 5. paracolpos; 6. clips where the cardinal ligament has been resected at the pelvic wall; 7. medial pedicle of the cardinal ligament; 8. uterine artery pedicle.
(From Burghardt E, Webb MJ, Monaghan JM, Kindermann G. Surgical Gynecologic Oncology. © Georg Thieme Verlag, 1993, with permission.)

tract infections in patients with indwelling catheters or residual urine, but do promote the development of resistant microorganisms. Stress incontinence after radical hysterectomy can be difficult to treat [27]. A short, scarred vagina with little mobility makes colposuspension difficult and the likelihood of postoperative voiding dysfunction is considerable. Periurethral injectables may be helpful in this setting.

Ureterovaginal and vesicovaginal fistulas are rare but should mentioned before surgery. In a review of 7,473 patients who underwent radical hysterectomy without adjuvant radiotherapy, the incidence of ureterovaginal and vesicovaginal fistulas was 2% and 0.9%, respectively [32]. Fistulas seem to be more common in patients undergoing aggressive procedures because of large tumours. Fistulas are commonly preceded by temperature spikes between the fifth and tenth postoperative days. Ureterovaginal fistulas can resolve after antegrade or retrograde stenting. The patient should be followed to rule out ureteral stenosis and obstruction.

Febrile morbidity occurs in 25% to 50% of patients after radical hysterectomy, depending on which definition is used. The most common causes are urinary tract infections, subclinical emboli, pulmonary atalectasis, wound infections, pelvic infections, haematomas or deep vein thrombosis. Pneumonia has become rare with routine respiratory care and early mobilisation.

Lymphocysts after radical hysterectomy appear to be less common if the pelvic peritoneum is left open. However, lymphocysts were rarely a clinical problem even when we closed the peritoneum; most were incidental findings in computed tomography [24]. On occasion lymphocysts can cause febrile morbidity, ureteral obstruction, and pelvic vein thrombosis. Treatment options include transabdominal or transvaginal aspiration and drainage. Aspirated fluid should be sent for cytology.

Intraoperative haemorrhage due to vascular lesions is uncommon. While arterial bleeding is usually relatively straightforward, lacerations of major veins can produce life-threatening haemorrhage that can be difficult to control. The surgeon should be familiar with fundamental vascular surgery techniques and should be able to close holes in major veins. Metal haemoclips are often useful; sometimes vascular sutures are required.

Damage to the obturator or genitofemoral nerve can occur during pelvic lymphadenectomy. The obturator nerve supplies the abductor muscles of the lower extremity. Damage to or division of the nerve causes weakness of these muscle groups. If the nerve is cut it should be sutured; regeneration after suturing is possible. If the nerve cannot be sutured, the patient should be referred for physical therapy to strengthen the compensatory muscles. Loss of the genitofemoral nerve leads to impaired sensation on the anterior and inner aspect of the thigh. Too deep retractor blades, particularly in thin patients, can cause presssure on and damage to the femoral nerve under the iliopsoas muscle. Typically patients with femoral nerve paresis have difficulty walking and climbing stairs or impaired sensation on the anterior aspect of the thigh, knee and inner aspect of the calf. Pressure damage to the femoral nerve takes months to resolve. The patient should be referred for physical therapy promptly.

Intraoperative deaths at radical hysterectomy have become very rare. Advances in surgery and perioperative care have reduced the mortality rate to 0.6% [32].

Results of surgical treatment and prognostic factors

The survival of patients after radical hysterectomy with pelvic lymphadenectomy is associated with risk factors identified at multivariate analyses.

■ Tumour size

Few authors have analysed survival according to tumour size or tumour volume [4, 5, 8]. Tumour volume is best measured in serial histologic sections of the uterus. Survival rates decrease with increasing tumour size, independently of other risk factors *(table I)*. Preoperative magnetic resonance imaging also provides reliable measurements of tumour volume [8] *(table II)*.

In a prospective Gynecologic Oncology Group study of 645 patients, the disease-free survival of patients with tumours less than 3 cm diameter was 85% compared with 68% for those with larger tumours [10].

Table I. 5-year survival according to tumour volume as measured in the surgical specimen (modified from Burghardt et al [51]).

Tumour volume	N	5 year survival
< 2.5 cm³	329	91 %
2.5 - 10 cm³	345	79%
> 10-50 cm³	330	70%

Table II. 5-year survival according to tumour volume measured pre-operatively by magnetic resonance imaging (modified from Winter [37]).

Tumour volume	N	5 year survival
< 10 cm³	42	95%
10 - 30 cm³	38	71%
> 30 cm³	37	64%

Table III. 5-year survival according to FIGO stage and lymph node status (modified from Benedet et al [2])

Stage	Negative nodes		Positive nodes	
	N	5 year survival	N	5 year survival
IB	1758	91%	467	66%
IIA	183	81%	84	55%
IIB	315	77%	165	46%

Table IV. 5-year survival according to number of positive lymph nodes (modified from Burghardt [3, 4]).

No of pos. nodes	N	5 year survival
0	256	89%
1	53	70%
2-3	60	62%
>4	51	37%

■ Lymph node status

The status of the lymph nodes is associated with tumour characteristics as well as with surgical and histologic characteristics. A number of authors have shown that the rate of pelvic node involvement is strongly associated with the size of the tumour [4].

Sampling or staging lymphadenectomies yield fewer pelvic lymph nodes than systematic attempts to remove the lymphatic tissue as completely as possible. The technique of histologic processing of the lymphatic tissue obtained at lymphadenectomy also affects the detection of node involvement. Processing the tissue en bloc in serial sections will detect more metastases than conventional histology.

The survival of patients with negative lymph nodes is significantly better than that of those with node involvement *(table III)*. Survival is also associated with the number of positive nodes, the number of positive node groups, and the size of the nodal metastases *(table IV, V, VI)*.

Table V. 5-year survival according to number of positive node groups (modified from Burghardt [3, 4])

No of positive node groups*	N	5 year survival
0	256	89%
1	76	70%
2	44	53%
3-7	44	39%

* Node groups: external iliac, common iliac, subaortic, obturator, presacral.

Table VI. 5-year survival according to size of lymph node metastases (modified from Burghardt [3, 4])

Size of node metastases	N	5 year survival
0*	260	90%
< 2 mm	35	68%
2-10 mm	47	59%
10-20 mm	58	54%
> 20 mm	20	39%

* Negative lymph nodes.

The rate of para-aortic node involvement increases with the number of positive pelvic nodes. In cervical cancer, para-aortic node involvement in patients with negative pelvic nodes ("skip" lesions) is very unusual. The survival rate of patients with positive para-aortic nodes is 20% to 40% [17, 31]. In a series of 90 patients who underwent radical hysterectomy with systematic pelvic and para-aortic lymphadenectomy, 17 patients had positive para-aortic nodes. After adjuvant treatment with carboplatin and bleomycin the 5-year survival rate of these patients was 60% [38]. These results suggest a benefit of lymphadenectomy, even in patients with positive para-aortic nodes.

Biopsy of the scalene lymph nodes should be considered in patients with positive para-aortic nodes because about 30% of these patients will have scalene node involvement.

■ Clinical staging

Clinical staging has a large subjective component. In the current 1994 FIGO staging system stage, IB1 tumours comprise lesions with a wide range of sizes and prognoses. Because tumour size correlates strongly with the rate of node involvement, survival rates of over 90% can be achieved in collectives with a rate of node involvement of 10% to 14% [3, 37]. If stage IB1 includes tumours with a rate of node involvement of 20% or more, survival rates are around 80% *(table VII)*. Increasing the surgical radicality seems to improve the results [21].

Only at a few centres is stage IIB disease, in which the rate of node metastases is 35% to 45%, treated with surgery *(table VIII)*. However, appropriately radical surgery is associated with survival rates of about 75%, which do not differ significantly from that of patients with stage IB disease *(table VIII)*. Sardi et al [30] reported that neoadjuvant platinum-based chemotherapy increased survival rates to 80%, as compared with 54% after surgery only.

■ Parametrial involvement

Histologically confirmed parametrial involvement is associated with a marked increase in the rate of pelvic lymph node involvement *(table IX)*. Tumour invasion of the vascular

Table VII. Survival and rates of lymph node involvement in published series of patients with FIGO stage Ib cervical cancer.

Study	No of patients	5 year survival	Positive nodes
Inoue & Okumura 1984 [15]	362	94%	13%
Hoyer 1990 [14]	115	95%	14%
Kjorstad et al 1983 [16]	612	81%	23%
Martimbeau 1978 [20]	353	82%	24%
Burghardt 1993 [3]	163	82%	31%

Table VIII. Survival and rates of lymph node involvement in published series of FIGO stage IIb cervical cancer.

Study	No of patients	5 year survival	Positive nodes
Inoue & Okumura 1983 [15]	223	78%	39%
Friedberg & Beck 1989 [12]	162	77%*	35%
Burghardt 1993 [3]	249	76%	45%

* Histological stage.

Table IX. 5-year survival according to involvement of the transitional zone of the cervix (modified from Burghardt [3, 4])

Transitional Zone	N	5 year survival
Not involved	234	83%
Involved	186	70%

transitional zone between the stroma of the cervix and the looser connective tissue of the parametrium has been made responsible for the rapid tumour spread.

■ Vascular space involvement

The prognostic significance of lymphatic space involvement is somewhat controversial [4, 8]. Some authors have reported a 5-year survival rate of 50% to 70% for patients with lymph vascular space involvement, compared with 90% for patients without invasion. Others have not been able to confirm the significance of lymph vascular space invasion after controlling for other risk factors. In invasive cervical cancers, lymph vascular space invasion is correlated with tumour size. The rate of pelvic lymph node involvement is higher in patients with lymph vascular space invasion than in patients without invasion. Lymph vascular space invasion seems to be more a risk factor for pelvic lymph node involvement than an independent prognostic factor for survival. Invasion of blood vessels has been associated with a significantly worse prognosis than invasion of lymphatic channels. Baltzer et al [1] reported 31% survival for patients with blood vessel invasion as opposed to 70% for those with lymphatic channel involvement.

References

[1] Baltzer J, Lohe KJ, Koepke W, Zander J. Histologic criteria for the prognosis in patients with operated squamous cell carcinoma of the cervix. *Gynecol Oncol* 1982 ; 13 : 184-194

[2] Benedet J, Odicino F, Maisonneuve P, Severl G, Creasman W, Shepherd J et al. Carcinoma of the cervix uteri. *J Epidemiol Biostat* 1998 ; 3 : 5-34

[3] Burghardt E. Cervical cancer: results. In : Burghardt E, Webb MJ, Monaghan JM, Kindermann G eds. Surgical gynecologic oncology. Stuttgart : Thieme, 1993 : 302-315

[4] Burghardt E. Prognostic factors of cervical cancer. In : Burghardt E, Webb MJ, Monaghan JM, Kindermann G eds. Surgical gynecologic oncology. Stuttgart : Thieme, 1993 : 315-323

[5] Burghardt E, Baltzer J, Tulusan AH, Haas J. Results of surgical treatment of 1028 cervical cancers studied with volumetery. *Cancer* 1992 ; 70 : 648-655

[6] Burghardt E, Haas J, Girardi F. The significance of the parametrium in the operative treatment of cervical cancer. *Baillière's Clin Obstet Gynaecol* 1988 ; 2 : 879-888

[7] Burghardt E, Winter R. Radical abdominal hysterectomy. In : Burghardt E, Webb MJ, Monaghan JM, Kindermann G eds. Surgical gynecologic oncology. Stuttgart : Thieme, 1993 : 290-293

[8] Burghardt E, Winter R, Tamussino K. Diagnosis and treatment of cervical cancer. *Crit Rev Oncol Hematol* 1994 ; 17 : 181-231

[9] Chamber SK, Chambers JT, Holm C, Peschel RE, Schwartz PE. Sequelae of lateral ovarian transposition un unirradiated cervical cancer patients. *Gynecol Oncol* 1990 ; 39 : 155-159

[10] Delgado G, Bundy B, Zaino R, Sevin BU, Creasman WT, Major F. Prospective surgical-pathological study of disease free interval in patients with stage Ib squamous cell carcinoma of the cervix: a gynecologic oncology group study. *Gynecol Oncol* 1990 ; 38 : 352-357

[11] Ellsworth LR, Allen HH, Nisker JA. Ovarian function after radical hysterectomy for stage IB carcinoma of the cervix. *Am J Obstet Gynecol* 1983 ; 145 : 185-188

[12] Friedberg V, Beck T. Ergebnisse operativer Therapie des Zervixkarzinoms im Stadium IIb. *Geburtsh Frauenheilk* 1989 ; 49 : 782-786

[13] Girardi F, Lichtenegger W, Tamussino K, Haas J. The importance of parametrial lymph nodes in the treatment of cervical cancer. *Gynecol Oncol* 1989 ; 34 : 206-211

[14] Hoyer M, Ljungstroem B, Nygland M, Jakobsen A. Radical hysterectomy in cervical carcinoma stage Ib. *Eur J Gynecol Oncol* 1990 ; 11 : 13-17

[15] Inoue T, Okumura M. Prognostic significance of parametrial extension in patients with cervical carcinoma stage Ib, IIa, IIb: a study of 628 cases treated by radical hysterectomy and lymphadenectomy with/or without postoperative irradiation. *Cancer* 1984 ; 54 : 1714-1719

[16] Kjörstad KE, Martimbeau P, Iversen T. Stage Ib carcinoma of the cervix at the Norwegian Radium Hospital: results and complications. *Gynecol Oncol* 1983 ; 15 : 42-47

[17] La Polla JP, Schlaerth JB, Gaddis O, Morrow CP. The influence of surgical staging on the evaluation and treatment of patients with cervical carcinoma. *Gynecol Oncol* 1986 ; 24 : 194-206

[18] Latzko W, Schiffmann J. Klinisches und anatomisches zur Radikaloperation des Gebärmutterhalskrebses. *Zentralbl Gynäkol* 1919 ; 34 : 689-719

[19] Lawton FG, Hacker NF. Surgery for invasive gynecologic cancer in an elderly female population. *Obstet Gynecol* 1990 ; 76 : 287-289

[20] Martimbeau PW, Kjorstad K, Kolstad P. Stage Ib carcinoma of the cervix at the Norwegian Radium Hospital 1968-1970: results of treatment and major complications. *Am J Obstet Gynecol* 1978 ; 131 : 389-394

[21] Monaghan JM, Irland D, Mor-Yosef S, Pearson SE, Lopes A, Sinha DP. Role of centralizazion of surgery in stage Ib carcinoma of the cervix: a review of 498 cases. *Gynecol Oncol* 1990 ; 37 : 206-209

[22] Owens S, Roberts WS, Fiorica JV, Hoffman MS, La Polla JP, Cavanagh D. Ovarian management at the time of radical hysterectomy for cancer of the cervix. *Gynecol Oncol* 1989 ; 35 : 349-351

[23] Peham H, Amreich J. Gynäkologische Operationstechnik. Berlin : S. Karger, 1930

[24] Petru E, Tamussino K, Lahousen M, Winter R, Pickel H, Haas J. Pelvic and paraaortic lymphocysts after radical surgery because of cervical and ovarian cancer. *Am J Obstet Gynecol* 1989 ; 161 : 937-941

[25] Piver MS, Rutledge F, Smith JP. Five classes of extended hysterectomy for women with cervical cancer. *Obstet Gynecol* 1974 ; 44 : 265-272

[26] Potish RA, Twiggs LB, Okagaki T, Prem KA, Adcock LL. Therapeutic implications of the natural history of advanced cervical cancer as defined by pretreatment surgical staging. *Cancer* 1985 ; 56 : 956-960

[27] Ralph G, Tamussino K. Surgical treatment of stress incontinence after radical hysterectomy. *Int Urogynecol J* 1992 ; 3 : 26-29

[28] Ralph G, Tamussino K, Lichtenegger W. Urological complications after radical abdominal hysterectomy with or without radiotherapy for cervical cancer. *Arch Gynecol Obstet* 1990 ; 248 : 61-65

[29] Ralph G, Winter R, Michelitsch L, Tamussino K. Radicality of parametrial resection and dysfunction of the lower urinary tract after radical hysterectomy. *Eur J Gynecol Oncol* 1991 ; 12 : 27-30

[30] Sardi JE, Sananes CE, Giaroli AA, Bermudez A, Ferreira MH, Soderini AH et al. Neoadjuvant chemotherapy in cervical carcinoma Stage IIb: a randomized controlled trial. *Int J Gynecol Cancer* 1998 ; 8 : 441-450

[31] Sevin BU, Averette HE. Staging laparotomy and radical hysterectomy for cancer of the cervix. *Baillière's Clin Obstet Gynaecol* 1988 ; 2 : 761-768

[32] Shingleton HM, Orr JW Jr. Recurrent cancer: exenterative surgery. In : Shingleton HM, Orr JW Jr eds. Cancer of the cervix. Philadelphia : JB Lippincott, 1995 : 259-321

[33] Tamussino K, Winter R, Lang PF. The cardinal ligament: surgical anatomy and resection. *CME Gynecol Oncol* 1997 ; 2 : 265-271

[34] Wertheim E. Zur Frage der Radikaloperation beim Uteruskrebs. *Arch Gynäkol* 1900 ; 61 : 627-668

[35] Winter R. Lymphademectomy. In : Burghardt E, Webb MJ, Monaghan JM, Kindermann G eds. Surgical gynecologic oncology. Stuttgart : Thieme, 1993 : 281-290

[36] Winter R. Radical surgery of the vaginal cuff after hysterectomy. In : Burghardt E, Webb MJ, Monaghan JM, Kindermann G eds. Surgical gynecologic oncology. Stuttgart : Thieme, 1993 : 295-297

[37] Winter R, Lahousen M, Haas J. Surgical treatment of stage Ib2 cervical cancer. *J Gynecol Tech* 1996 ; 2 : 207-212

[38] Winter R, Lahousen M, Haas J, Burghardt E. Long-term survival of patients with paraaortic metastasis. [abstract]. Presented at the 46th annual meeting of the Society of Pelvic Surgeons, Lexington Kentucky, October 11-13, 1995

Chapter 8

Radiotherapy for stage I-II cervical cancer

Erik Van Limbergen, Christine Haie-Meder

E Van Limbergen, Associate Professor in Radiation Oncology, U.Z. Gasthuisberg, Herestraat 49, Leuven, Belgium.
C Haie-Meder, Head of the Department of Brachytherapy, Institut Gustave Roussy, Villejuif, France.

Radiotherapy for stage I-II cervical cancer

E Van Limbergen, C Haie-Meder

Abstract. — *Stage Ib and proximal IIb cervical cancer can be cured either by radical surgery or radiotherapy. These two procedures are equally effective as concern local control and survival, as has been demonstrated in several retrospective and randomised studies. Radiotherapy is feasible and effective in almost all patients, resulting in 5-year survival rates of 78% to 91%, as compared to 54% to 90% after radical surgery for early stage cervical cancer. Primary radical surgery affords, in contrast to primary radiotherapy, the opportunity to use pathological findings to select patients for adjuvant treatment. However, to achieve the reported cure rates, adjuvant treatment is used in about 50% of patients having tumours of less than 4 cm and in about 80% of those with tumours larger than 4 cm, because of positive nodes, or positive or close section margins.*

With modern techniques, complication rates after primary radical radiotherapy have been shown to be significantly lower than after primary surgery. The highest complication rates are seen when surgery and radiotherapy are combined. However, in some situations where preoperative radiotherapy or brachytherapy is adapted to surgery, particularly in terms of dose and irradiated volumes, severe complications can be observed in less than 5% of the patients.

The choice of treatment is not easy and will depend largely on the policy of the institution, as well as the gynaecologists or radiation oncologists involved. The age (gonadal sparing) and the general health (operability) of the patient, as well as the need for postoperative irradiation after a primary surgical approach, may have an impact on the final decision.

Keywords: primary radical radiotherapy, brachytherapy, operability.

Radiotherapy indications in stage I and stage II cervical cancer

Radiotherapy (RT) is used either in a radical radiation treatment protocol with external beam radiotherapy and brachytherapy, or in a combined protocol of surgery and preoperative or postoperative irradiation.

Uterovaginal brachytherapy is an essential tool in radiation treatment for cervical carcinoma, delivering high central pelvic doses to the tumour while sparing to some degree the surrounding critical organs such as the bladder, rectum and small bowel. Brachytherapy is delivered at a continuous low dose rate (LDR) or pulsed dose rate (PDR) or in fractionated sessions at a high dose rate (HDR). Brachytherapy alone can be indicated in stage Ia, where no treatment of the lymph nodes is indicated. This stage, however, is usually treated by surgery alone, seldom to be completed by postoperative vaginal brachytherapy in case of positive vaginal section margins.

For limited disease (stages Ib and IIa) and stage IIb, proximal brachytherapy is used for definite radiation treatment in combination with external beam irradiation (EBRT) to the pelvis, or as a preoperative modality in combination with radical surgery.

In radical radiotherapy, pelvic EBRT is used to shrink bulky tumours and to improve the local anatomy so that the high dose portion of the intracavitary dose distribution can adequately cover the tumour extension. EBRT also sterilises parametrial and nodal disease that lies beyond the reach of the uterovaginal application.

In a postoperative setting, pelvic EBRT is performed, according to pathological findings, to sterilise microscopic pelvic disease in high risk patients, while vaginal brachytherapy may be indicated in selected cases. These postoperative indications are discussed in chapter 9.

Radiotherapy techniques

- External beam radiotherapy: target volume, technique, dose and fractionation

Pelvic EBRT

The target volume for pelvic EBRT encompasses the cervix and the tumour extensions into the uterus, vagina and parametria. Depending on the stage and the tumoural lower limit, the upper two-thirds of the vagina or the entire vagina are included. It also covers the draining lymph nodes at risk: parametrial, internal obturator and internal iliac, external iliac, common iliac and presacral nodes down to the S2-S3 junction.

Due to the diameter of the patients at the level of the pelvis, EBRT should be delivered by mega-voltage photon beams (10 MV – 20 MV) by a multiportal technique. Lower energies may cause excessive subcutaneous fibrosis and higher rectal or bladder doses. Usually, a 4 field box technique is used (2 opposed anteroposterior fields and 2 lateral fields) to reduce gastrointestinal and bladder morbidity *(fig 1)*. The fields are individually shaped so that the target is adequately covered while other pelvic contents that are not at risk for recurrence are blocked out. Standard fields for pelvic irradiation usually extend from the L4-L5 interspace or the middle of L5 to the bottom of the foramen obturatorium or tuber ischiadium. A 1.5 to 2 cm safety margin lateral to the pelvic rim is usually sufficient to cover the lymph node areas *(fig 2)*. Standard lateral fields extend anteriorly from the pubic bone to the G2-G3 interspace posteriorly *(fig 3)*.

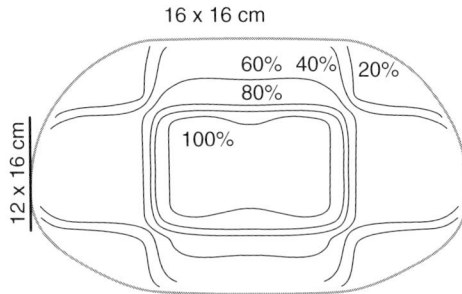

Figure 1. *Field box technique for external beam radiotherapy in cervical cancer. This technique allows sparing of the anterior (bladder and small bowel) and posterior (rectosigmoid) parts of the pelvis.*

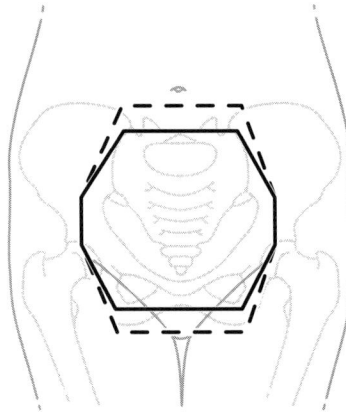

Figure 2. *AP-PA view of pelvic EBRT field for cervical cancer stage I-II, used in radical RT in combination with uterovaginal brachytherapy, or post-operatively after surgery in high risk patients (larger fields) or intermediate risk patients (smaller fields).*

However, it has been demonstrated repeatedly that with standard fields the target may be outside the treated volume in up to 25% of cases [12, 35]. Most of the time, this occurs at the posterior border of the lateral fields. Therefore, it is strongly recommended to use CT or MRI to locate the target correctly in the pelvis and to adapt the borders of the radiation fields to the individual patient. This not only prevents geographical misses, but also allows reducing unnecessary irradiation of parts of the bladder and small bowel [12].

AP-PA fields can be used when high-energy photons are available or when there is uterosacral lymph node involvement. Some institutes use AP-PA fields with central shielding for the bladder and rectum, thus allowing higher centropelvic doses to be delivered by the uterovaginal brachytherapy. In that case, the first uterovaginal insertion is already performed at 20 Gy pelvic EBRT, with further EBRT performed with a central block in place.

Construction of the ideal midline block has been a source of controversy. Some institutions use rectangular midline blocks which are 3-5 cm wide, covering the position of the intrauterine brachytherapy. Others use standard small, medium, and large step

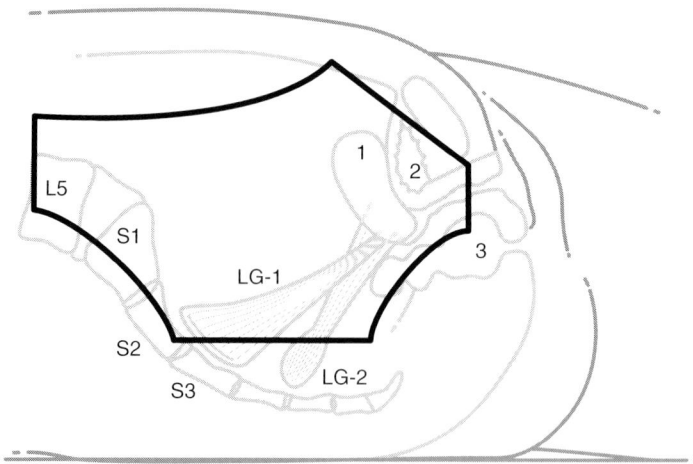

Figure 3. *Lateral view of pelvic EBRT field with individual shaping of field margins, based on sectional imaging with CT. 1. Uterus; 2. bladder; 3. rectum.*

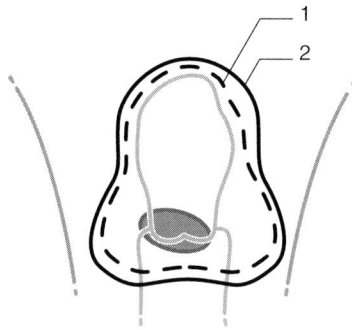

Figure 4. *Pear-shaped isodose distribution of uterovaginal brachytherapy. 1. Target volume; 2. treatment volume.*

wedge blocks adapted to the ovoids. Other institutions have developed customised midline blocks based on the isodose distribution of the initial implant *(fig 4)* or even several stepwise decreasing isodoses. Midline blocks should always be constructed and placed with extreme care to avoid under-dosing the tumour in the lateral parametria or over-dosing the critical central structures. Eifel et al [7] detected an increase in complications in patients with midline blocks 4 cm wide used throughout the course of EBRT. Because the ureters are typically 2-3 cm from the midline, the increase in ureteral complications seen in this series was due to an overlap between the EBRT fields and the high-dose region of the intracavitary implant. Eifel recommends a margin of 0.5 cm lateral to the lateral ovoid surface to determine the width of the midline block so as to protect the implanted volume.

Many institutions prefer to deliver 40-50 Gy of EBRT in 1.8-2 Gy per fraction to the entire pelvis, on the assumption that it is advantageous to deliver a homogeneous distribution to this region at risk for microscopic disease, obtaining maximal shrinkage of central disease before intracavitary irradiation. Accordingly, the brachytherapy dose is decreased to respect normal tissue tolerance. However, larger volumes of the bladder, rectum and small bowel are treated by this technique.

Depending on the stage and treatment protocol, the total dose delivered by external irradiation may thus range between 20 Gy to 55 Gy, taking into account the contribution of brachytherapy. In general, the external irradiation dose increases with the tumour stage to deliver adequate doses to the latero-pelvic region.

In case of chemoradiation, for instance in combination with weekly CDDP 40 mg/m^2, the total dose is reduced by $\pm$ 10% (i.e. 45 Gy in 1.8-2 Gy per fraction), to compensate for the 10% increase in late gut toxicity (dose modifying factor 1.1).

It is advised to treat all fields daily.

Boost to pelvic nodes

An additional dose of 5-10 Gy after the 45-50 Gy pelvic irradiation may be delivered to areas of macroscopic disease with an anteroposterior (AP) or 4 field technique, or conformal radiotherapy, depending on the volume and the localisation of the involved nodes.

■ Brachytherapy

Uterovaginal brachytherapy

Uterovaginal brachytherapy offers the possibility of delivering high doses to the central pelvis, while sparing the surrounding normal tissues at risk for complications. By applying an intrauterine source carrier and paracervical intravaginal sources, an almost pear-shaped isodose pattern is delivered to the target volume, which includes the cervix uteri, the proximal third of the vagina and the proximal third of the parametria (fig 4). Doses to the bladder and rectum are kept under the normal tissue tolerance level, because of the exponential fall of the dose with distance from the sources.

Different systems are available, which may vary both in the applicator design and the loading pattern. The intra-uterine applicators, often called "tandem applicators", exist in various lengths. They may be straight or curved to various angles to allow for different degrees of anteversion of the uterus. For the intravaginal sources, ovoids with caps of different sizes exist (half, small, medium, large) to adapt to the available space in the upper vagina (fig 5A, B). Different sizes of ring applicators may also be used (fig 5C). It is also possible to fabricate individual mould applicators, which are adapted to individual variations of local anatomy and tumour extensions [11]. Especially in non-standard conditions, these light-weight and individually designed applicators have the advantage of optimally adapted positioning of the intravaginal sources (fig 5D).

All of the modern after-loading applicators have fixation systems to immobilise the chosen spacing of the intravaginal source carriers as well as the protruding and angling of the intrauterine sources according to the ovoids. All these systems exist for manual or remote controlled LDR, PDR or HDR after-loading systems with cesium, cobalt, or iridium sources.

The applicators are usually inserted under general anaesthesia. A Foley catheter is placed in the bladder. The fixation balloon is filled with 7-cc contrast medium, which allows marking the base of the bladder for dosimetry (fig 6).

After hysterometry and dilatation of the cervix, an intrauterine source carrier of the appropriate length is inserted. Then the vaginal source carrier(s), either two ovoid type

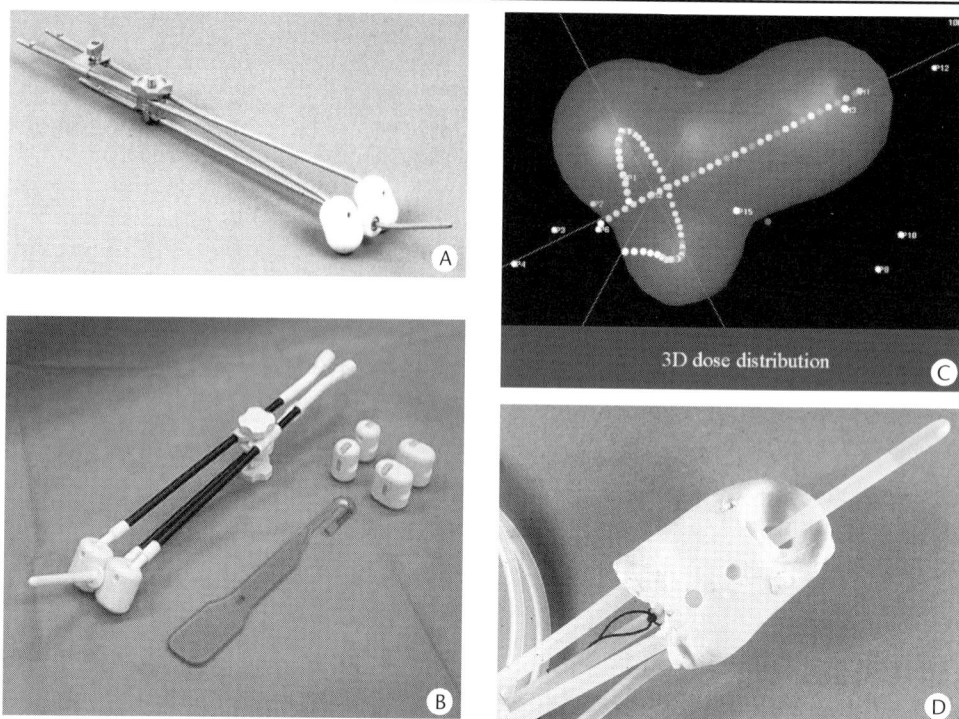

Figure 5. *Applicators used with uterovaginal bracytherapy in cervical cancer.*
   A. Fletcher type with tandem and ovoids.
   B. NMR compatible carbon applicator.
   C. Ring applicator.
   D. Individual vaginal mould applicator.

applicators or a vaginal ring applicator of the appropriate size (or an individually fabricated vaginal mould), is inserted. It is very important to carefully adjust the position of the intrauterine source in relation to the vaginal sources, and to fix the chosen positions. Vaginal gauze packing, special retractors *(fig 5B)* or the individual mould *(fig 5D)* help to push the bladder and rectal wall away from the sources. Finally, a rectal catheter is inserted. This allows rectal filling with a contrast medium/air mixture at the time of the localisation films for opacification of the rectal walls.

After the application, orthogonal X-rays are taken from the implant for dosimetric calculations. Sectional imaging with CT, ultrasound or MRI is useful to provide additional information on target delineation and the exact positions of the bladder and rectal walls relative to the sources *(fig 7)*. However, metallic applicators may cause important artefacts on CT and are not suitable for MR imaging. Special non-metallic (carbon) MRI compatible applicators must be inserted for this purpose *(fig 5B)*.

The duration of the application is calculated according to the treatment planning system.

As has been developed by the Manchester school, the dose can be prescribed to point A, which is a point situated 2 cm lateral from the central source and 2 cm above the vaginal fornix *(fig 8)*. The dose to point A, however, is not sufficient to characterise the parameters of a brachytherapy application, especially in terms of complication risk assessment. Moreover, the definition of point A is not totally standardised and, with the

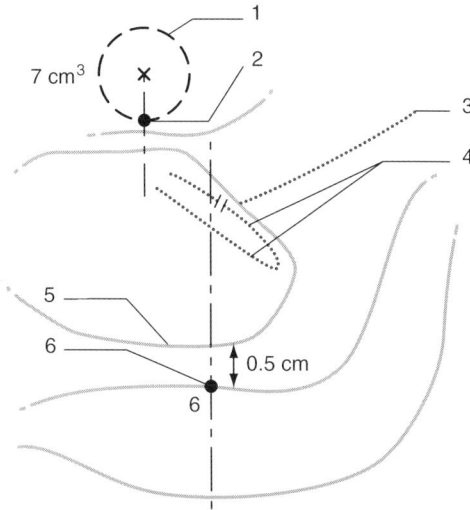

Figure 6. *ICRU bladder and rectum reference points to determine the dose to critical organs in uterovaginal brachytherapy for cervical cancer. 1. Balloon 7 cm²; 2. bladder reference point; 3. intrauterine source; 4. intravaginal sources; 5. vaginal posterior wall; 6. rectal reference point.*

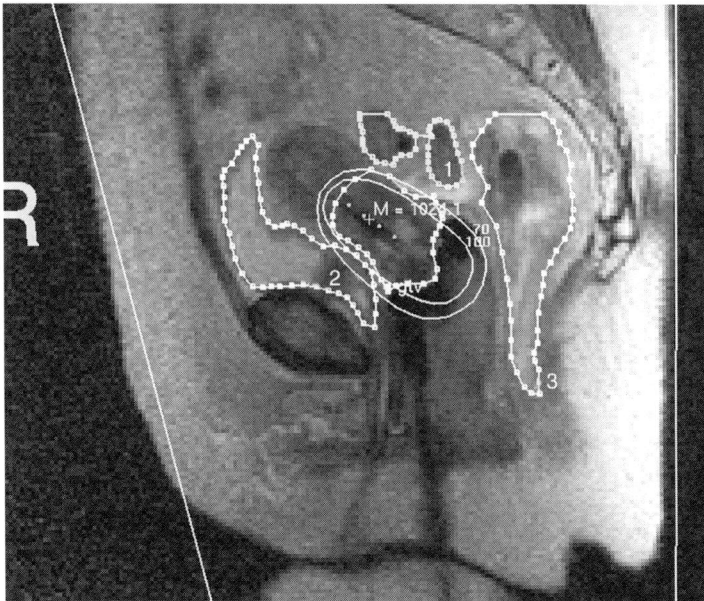

Figure 7. *Use of MRI sectional imaging to delineate the target volume for brachytherapy and the position of surrounding critical organs (bladder, rectum, small bowel) in three dimensions.*

rapid dose fall off, may vary from one institution to the other. The relation of a given dose distribution pattern according to point A is only valid for a certain geometry and

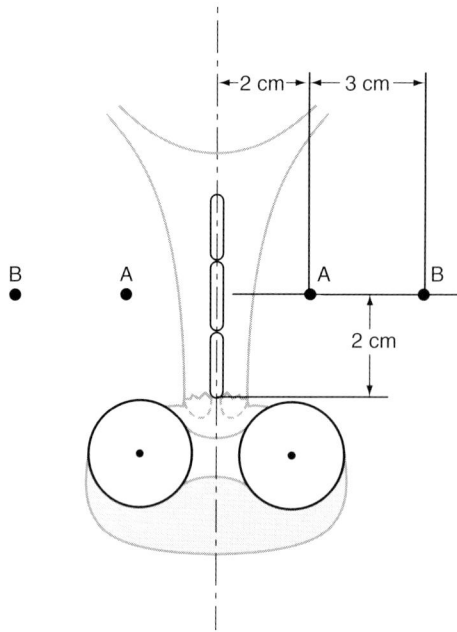

Figure 8. *Manchester Points A and B, situated left and right, 2 and 5 cm to the intrauterine flange, 2 cm above the vaginal fornices. Since dose distribution around the sources depends on source lengths, spacing and relative loading pattern (uterine versus vaginal), the dose to Point A gives only partial information on dose distribution.*

loading pattern. Different geometries and loading patterns lead to different pear or banana shaped isodoses, although they may deliver the same dose to point A.

It is up to the clinician to determine the source lengths, source positioning and application time that will deliver the desired dose distribution to the target volume and to the critical organs. This may be according to a standard protocol developed at different institutions or highly adapted to the individual anatomy, tumour extension and treatment strategy (preoperative versus radical RT), doses of EBRT and brachytherapy dose rates.

For reasons of comparability, the ICRU [17] recommends to report the characteristics of a brachytherapy application by the following items: applicator and source type used, the total reference air kerma, the volume of the 60 Gy reference isodose, the doses to critical organs such as bladder, rectum, pelvic walls and pelvic lymph nodes.

Doses to point A, delivered by external beam and low dose rate brachytherapy usually vary from 65 to 75 Gy for small tumours and 70 to 90 Gy for larger tumours [21, 29]. For PDR or HDR brachytherapy, it is recommended to give the radiobiological equivalent doses to the target volume and to the critical organs, taking into account the different impacts of dose rate, fraction size and treatment duration. In any case, the individual HDR fraction sizes should be less than 7.5 Gy due to reports of higher toxicity with fractions sized > 7.5 Gy [25].

Interstitial brachytherapy

In patients with a normal anatomy, the placement of interstitial needles is seldom required in brachytherapy for early stage cervix cancer. However, in selected cases of cervical stump carcinoma or in case of an inaccessible vagina, a transvaginal or transperineal interstitial approach might be considered to perform a centropelvic brachytherapy.

Results

■ Radical RT treatment

In the 1998 FIGO annual report [8] concerning patients treated between 1990-92 by definitive radiotherapy, the overall survival at 5 years reported for stage Ib (1,194 patients) was 72.2%, for stage IIa (422 patients) 64.6% and for IIb (1,784 patients) 63.7%. These results are similar to those published for radical surgery, although the patients selected for surgery are usually younger, less obese and in a better general state of health. In the annual report (1998) for patients treated between 1990-92 by surgery alone (mostly better risk patients), the overall survival at 5 years was 90% for stage Ib (1,287 patients), 66% for stage IIa (73 patients) and 80% for IIb (78 patients). For patients treated with surgery followed by radiotherapy (usually because of high risk features), the survival rate was 80.1% for Ib, 68.2% for IIa and 63.7% for IIb.

■ EBRT with LDR brachytherapy

An overview of the literature on recent large studies [16, 22, 29] shows an overall survival at 5 years between 80% and 89% with a pelvic failure rate between 7% and 12% in stage Ib (1,115 patients). In stage IIa (590 patients), the overall survival was between 70% and 85%, with a pelvic failure rate ranging from 8.5% to 19%. In stage IIb (667 patients), a survival rate between 72% and 76% and a pelvic failure of 20-23% were reported *(table I)*.

In a French collaborative study concerning 1,383 patients treated according to the Fletcher-Horiot method, a 5-year survival for stage Ib of 89%, stage IIa of 85%, and stage IIb of 76% was obtained, as well as local control rates for stage Ib of 93%, IIa of 88% and IIb of 78% [16]. These results are comparable to those published by Carlos Perez with a 5-year survival rate / local control of: 87% / 94% for 281 stage Ib, 73% / 88% for 88 stage IIa, and 68% / 83% for 252 stage IIb.

In a recent randomised trial [21], 343 patients with cervical cancer stage Ib - IIa were treated either with radical radiotherapy or colpohysterectomy and lymphadenectomy, followed by pelvic radiotherapy in a subgroup of patients with high risk for recurrence. This was the case in 54% of tumours less than 4 cm and in 84% of the patients with tumours larger than 4 cm because of positive nodes (25% - 31%) or positive or close section margins (45% - 67%).

At 5 years, the survival rates (83%) and recurrence free survival rates (76%) were identical in both radical radiotherapy and surgery (+ - adjuvant pelvic radiotherapy) arms. However, complication rates were dependent on the treatment received.

Results of radical radiotherapy are strongly dependent on the size of the tumour, rather than on the stage. Lowrey [22] reported a 10 year pelvic control rate of 81%-100% for stage Ib, IIa, and IIb for tumours smaller than 3 cm, 84%-88% if between 4 to 5 cm, and 60 to 76% if larger than 6 cm.

Table I. Results of radiotherapy for cervical cancer.

A) Stage Ib

	n	5 year Survival	5 year Local Control	Severe Complications
Horiot et al 1988 [16]	192 LDR	89 %	93 %	5 %
Perez et al 1991 [29]	281 LDR	87 %	94 %	5 %
Gerbaulet et al [11]	281 LDR preop	92 %	95 %	4.3 %
Lowrey 1992 [22]	130 LDR	95 %	92 %	3 %
Orton et al 1991 [25]	630 LDR	82.4 %		
Orton et al 1991 [25]	1327 HDR	82.7 %		
Landoni et al 1997 [21]	167 LDR*	83 %	84 %	

B) Stage IIa

	n	5 year Survival	5 year Local Control	Severe Complications
Horiot et al 1988 [16]	315 LDR	85 %	88 %	5 %
Perez et al 1991 [29]	88 LDR	73 %	88 %	9 %
Lowrey 1992 [22]	64 LDR	75 %	85 %	4 %
Gerbaulet et al 1992 [11]	See IIB*			
Orton et al 1991 [25]	See IIB*			

C) Stage IIb

	n	5 year Survival	5 year Local Control	Severe Complications
Horiot et al 1988 [16]	314 LDR	76 %	78 %	9 %
Perez et al 1991 [29]	252 LDR	68 %	83 %	11 %
Lowrey 1992 [22]	112 LDR	68 %	80 %	6 %
Gerbaulet et al 1992 [11]	149 preop LDR and surgery	78 %	79 %	6.7 %
Orton et al 1991 [25]	1271 LDR**	66.8 %		
Orton et al 1991 [25]	2891 HDR**	66.6 %		

* IIa included in Ib results
** IIA included in the IIb results

Landoni [21] reported 10% pelvic recurrences in stage Ib-IIa tumours less than 4 cm and 32% if larger than 4 cm.

EBRT with HDR brachytherapy

Several studies (including randomised and non-randomised prospective clinical trials, surveys of published studies, and meta-analysis) have compared results of LDR brachytherapy to HDR brachytherapy for cervical cancer; these have demonstrated comparable local control, survival and complication rates. In overviews by Fu and Phillips in 1990 [9] and Orton et al in 1991 [25], 5-year survival rates are about 90% in stage Ib and 60-70% in stage IIb.

A review of world literature by Fu et al [9] compared results in 1,764 HDR patients with 2,370 patients treated with LDR. They concluded that most of the non-randomised studies suggested similar survival and local control rates using fractionated remote after-loading HDR intracavitary brachytherapy combined with EBRT for carcinoma of the cervix, as compared to historical or concurrent LDR controls. Only two of the 10 institutions studied reported any significant differences in survival after LDR or HDR, and these showed improved survival with HDR.

Shigematsu et al [36] reported on 143 patients treated with HDR therapy compared to 106 patients treated with LDR for stage IIb and III disease. Superior local control was found for the HDR treatment arm. There was no difference in survival. However, the randomisation technique of the study has been criticised, since some patients randomised to LDR were actually treated with HDR (because of limited LDR availability or because many older patients were treated preferentially with HDR).

In a randomised trial reported by Patel [27], a total of 482 patients were randomised to receive either LDR brachytherapy at 0.55-0.65 Gy/h to point A, or 9.0-9.5 Gy/fraction with HDR. Early stage patients received intracavitary brachytherapy with doses of 75 Gy to point A in two fractions (LDR) or 38 Gy in four fractions (HDR) in addition to a midline blocked pelvic external beam of 35 Gy.

Orton et al [25] performed a meta-analysis of 17,068 patients treated with HDR and 5,666 with LDR. Published data and information derived from a mailed questionnaire were included. The overall 5-year survival rates were similar: 60.8% for HDR and 59.0% for LDR.

■ Preoperative radiosurgical combination in limited disease

In the annual FIGO report (1998) for patients treated between 1990-92 by preoperative external radiotherapy and/or intracavitary brachytherapy, the overall survival at 5 years for stage Ib (440 patients) was 84%, for stage IIa (80 patients) 80%, and for IIb (118 patients) 58%. In a series of 441 stage I and proximal stage II patients treated at the Institut Gustave Roussy, a 5-year survival rate of 87% and a pelvic failure rate of 5% were obtained.

■ Optimisation of radiotherapy

The success and complication rates of radiotherapy are dependent on the stage, radiation dose and volume treated. However, the dose delivery pattern over time, the haemoglobin levels during radiotherapy and the combination of radiation with chemotherapy also play an important role and may be optimised during treatment.

Time dose pattern

It has been repeatedly demonstrated in retrospective analyses [14, 30, 32] that a treatment duration longer than 52-60 days may result in worse local control rates and survival, as compared to treatment in shorter overall times. It is assumed that this worse local control is caused by accelerated tumour cell repopulation during protracted radiation. Girinsky et al [14] demonstrated, in a retrospective multivariate analysis of 386 stage IIb and III cervical cancers, a significant impact of total treatment time on local control ($P < 0.005$) and survival ($P < 0.001$). For each day beyond a total treatment time of 52 days, a reduction of 1% in the local control rate and survival was found. The same experience was reported by Petereit [32] in 209 stage I-IIIb patients showing a reduction of 0.7% in the local control rate and of 0.6% in survival for every additional treatment day over 55 days.

These data stress that radical radiotherapy, both EBRT and BT, should be given within a time period of 7 to 8 weeks. When LDR or PDR brachytherapy is performed after EBRT, it is recommended to minimise the treatment interval. If multiple insertions are planned or required, such as in HDR to avoid the detrimental effects of large fraction sizes to the critical organs, it is advised to interdigitate the applications during the EBRT. If the vaginal geometry is adequate, brachytherapy is started early in the course of EBRT. In large tumours where shrinkage of the tumour requires the whole EBRT series, it is advised to perform two implants per week to keep the total treatment time below 8 weeks.

Haemoglobin level

Decreased haemoglobin levels have been associated with decreased efficacy of radiotherapy in patients with cervical cancer. Anaemia may be caused by blood loss due to the primary tumour, previous surgery or by myelosuppression under chemotherapy.

In advanced cervical cancer, anaemia has been shown to be an independent prognostic factor for outcome after primary radiotherapy [2, 10, 13, 33].

In a multivariate analysis of 386 patients with advanced cervical cancer receiving radiotherapy, Girinsky et al [13] demonstrated that Hb values below 10 g/dL represent a significant negative prognosis factor. Even a single Hb value under 10 g/dL during radiotherapy had a negative effect on overall survival.

In another retrospective analysis, 162 patients with a tumour size of T ≥ 3 cm and Hb values less than 11 g/dL had a significantly worse relapse-free survival rate [33].

A randomised study by Bush et al [2] showed that a systematic increase of Hb value above 12.5 g/dL, which was achieved by blood transfusions, resulted in a significantly higher rate of local control, as compared to patients in the control arm. Similar results were also reported for the significance of pO_2 as a prognostic factor in other tumour entities. For this reason, it is strongly recommended to keep Hb during radiotherapy at levels of at least 12g/dL.

Role of concomitant chemotherapy

Several randomised studies have been carried out recently. Comparing concomitant chemotherapy with standard radiotherapy, they show a reduction in the risk of death by 30% to 50% for CDDP based chemotherapy combined with radiotherapy. The data show a statistically significant benefit from chemoradiation, particularly in early disease; this is less significant in patients with advanced stage III and IVa disease.

In the GOG 85 study [39], 386 patients with stage IIb, III and IVa were randomised to receive radiotherapy and chemotherapy: either hydroxyurea for 6 weeks, or hydroxyurea and 2 courses of CDDP and 5-FU. All the patients had negative cytological washings and negative para-aortic lymph nodes. The 3 year progression-free survival was 67% for those treated with CDDP-RT and 57% for the hydroxyurea RT group ($P = 0.03$)

In the GOG 120 study [34], 526 patients with stage IIb, III and IVa with negative para-aortic lymph nodes at para-aortic lymphadenectomy were randomised to either hydroxyurea 3g/m² twice weekly for six weeks, or hydroxyurea with 2 pulses of CDDP 50 mg/m² and 5-FU 4g/m² over 96 hours every 4 weeks. In a third arm, weekly CDDP at 40 mg/m² for 6 weeks was given. The 3 year progression-free survival for women treated with CDDP (arms 2 and 3) was 67% versus 47% in the hydroxyurea only arm ($P = 0.002$). Although the 2 CDDP containing schedules resulted in the same survival, toxicity was significantly lower in the weekly CDDP arm, with grade 3 and 4 acute toxicity twice as great in the hydroxyurea-CDDP arm.

In the GOG trial 123 [18], 374 women with bulky stage Ib (> 4 cm) and with normal para-aortic lymph nodes on CT or lymphangiography were randomised to radiotherapy or radiotherapy and weekly cisplatinum (40 mg/m²). At a median follow-up time of 36 months, 74% of those treated with RT alone and 83% of those treated with CDDP-RT were alive (overall survival $P = 0.008$), with a relative risk of death of 0.54 for the combination arm.

In the RTOG trial 9001 [24], 388 patients with stage Ib-IIa larger than 5 cm, or IIb, III, IVa cancers with negative para-aortic lymph nodes on lymphangiography or CT, were randomised to either extended field irradiation (pelvic + para-aortic) versus pelvic radiotherapy combined with 2 cycles of CDDP (75 mg/m²) and 5-FU (4g/m² over 96 hours) with a 3 week interval. The 5 year overall survival was 58% in the extended field RT arm, versus 73% in the arm with chemoradiation ($P = 0.004$), with a reduction of the mortality rate of 0.52 for the latter.

Complications

Complications may result from many treatment related factors, especially in cervical carcinoma where several types of treatment are frequently combined: surgery, brachytherapy, external beam radiotherapy, chemotherapy.

These complications may be acute or delayed; they can occur over an extremely variable period, from several days to several years after the end of treatment.

In addition, some complications may not be taken into account in statistics due to recurrence of the cancer or the premature death of the patient.

Evaluating the severity of complications may also be problematic, due to the element of subjectivity in their assessment. The evaluation system for complications developed by the RTOG covers all types of organs involved and is applicable to all treatment localisations; however, this scoring system is not specific for the complications of cervical carcinoma. Chassagne et al [4] have developed and published a glossary of complications which is more specific for cervical cancer and which makes it possible to compare different treatment modalities. This Franco-Italian glossary describes the complications affecting 14 organs and/or healthy tissues; their increasing severity is expressed by a scoring system graded 0 to 4. The use of this system proved to be reliable and reproducible for a randomised study comparing two radiotherapy dose rates, for which complications were one of the evaluation criteria [15]. This trial also showed that prospective registration is the ideal way to analyse complications. It is also necessary to study the evolution of complications: over the course of time, they may resolve, remain stable or become worse, and new complications may also occur.

It is then necessary to treat all of the registered data by means of an adequate statistical methodology which takes all of the parameters into account. Analysis of the prevalence appears to be the best adapted to the various situations [19]. This is based on a "life history model" where each patient moves between different states as a function of time and the occurrence and evolution of one or more complications. Of course, this model also takes into consideration a recurrence of the cancer and/or the death of the patient.

- ■ Complications of radiotherapy alone

In cercival carcinoma treated by radiotherapy alone, it is difficult to separate those complications caused by external radiation from those linked to brachytherapy. Data from the literature generally concern global evaluations of complications, which are most often studied in terms of their locations.

Frequency and location of complications

In a series published by Crook [6] which concerned 348 patients with stage I to III cancer, the glossary developed by Chassagne et al [4] was used. The complication rates were reported as 19.5% grade I, 19% grade 2, and 9.8% grade 3. Forty-eight percent of the grade 2 and 3 complications were rectal, 21% were urinary, and 15% rectosigmoid. In this study, no significant difference in the rate of complications appeared between stages I and II. These data have been recently updated and have confirmed the reliability of this glossary with an accurate correlation of morbidity and survival over time [11]. In the earlier series, the use of this glossary was limited in the grade 3 complication group which appeared to comprise an inhomogeneous cohort of patients. The scoring for grade 3 did not take into account complications with potential long-term detriment, so that a division into three subgroups was proposed.

In a study by Perez [28] concerning 811 patients, 10% developed a grade 2 complication and 8% a grade 3 complication. Of these, 8% of the patients had grade 2 or 3 gastrointestinal complications, and 5% grade 2 or 3 urinary complications. Five percent of the patients experienced grade 2 complications at another location, mainly vaginal stenoses. The frequency and severity of the complications appeared to be independant of the cancer stage.

A study by Sinistrero [37] concerned 215 patients with cancer stages I through III. Among them, 21.8% presented grade I complications, 5.5% had grade 2 complications and 5% grade 3 complications (only one patient had grade 4). Digestive system complications were the most frequent (58.3%), followed by urinary complications (29.1%) and others (12.5%).

Eifel published a study [7] of 1,784 patients with stage Ib. The rate of serious complications ($\geq$ 3) at five years was 9.3%. The risk of serious urinary complications was 0.7% per year for the first three years, then it decreased to 0.25% per year for the next 25 years. The risk of rectal complications was 1% per year for two years and then decreased to 0.06% per year between 2 and 25 years.

Time of occurrence

For the Crook study [6], the mean time for occurrence of rectal and rectosigmoid complications was 19 months and for urinary complications 28 months after the beginning of treatment. Grade 3 complications appeared in 64% of the cases before

24 months, and 82% after 36 months. These data were confirmed by Sinistrero [37] who noted that 8 out of 11 grade 3 complications occurred in the first 24 months following treatment; for all complications, regardless of grade, the average time of occurrence was 23 months. Eifel [7] insists on the necessity to closely monitor patients – although the majority of serious complications occur in the first 5 years, there is still a risk of later occurrence, which is estimated at 0.34% per year, resulting in an actuarial risk of major complications of 14.4% at 20 years.

Factors influencing the occurrence of complications

Previous pelvic surgery or inflammatory pelvic disease

In a study of 111 patients, Eifel [7] reports that the risk of fistulas is twice as high for patients having undergone a pretreatment laparotomy (5.2% versus 2.9%; $P = 0.007$), and the risk of small bowel obstruction is significantly higher in this same group of patients (14.5% versus 3.7% at 10 years; $P < 0.0001$). To the contrary, Perez [28, 29] found no correlation between these factors and the occurrence of complications. The dose is reduced by 5 to 10% in cases where there are risk factors of this type.

Age

Age is a more controversial factor. Lanciano [20], in his report on the "Patterns of Care Study", found that complications were more frequent in women less than 36 years old. Perez [28, 29] did not find any influence of age, but did mention a dose reduction on the order of 5 to 10% for women over 65.

Factors related to irradiation parameters

Total dose

Perez [28, 29] reported a rate of urinary or rectal complications which is significantly higher when the total dose to the bladder or rectum exceeded 80 Gy. Pourquier described twice as many urinary or rectosigmoid complications with doses higher than 75 to 80 Gy. Within the framework of the "Patterns of Care Study", Lanciano [20] recommends a point A dose of 85 Gy. In this same study, the risk of major complications was also linked to latero-pelvic doses higher than 50 Gy.

Volume and dose to critical organs

Crook [6] has established diagrams with 3 different zones according to low, moderate or high risks of complications, taking into account the volume irradiated and the dose to criticial organs such as the bladder or rectum. Used in a prospective manner, these factors helped to decrease the incidence of complications. Sinistrero [37] also found that the dose influenced complications, with a mean cumulative dose of 55.76 Gy for an absence of complications, of 61.82 Gy for grade 1 complications, 63 Gy for grade 2 complications and 73.7 Gy for grade 3 complications.

Perez [28, 29] insists on the importance of computerised tomography (CT scan) in the incidence of serious rectal or rectosigmoid complications (rates of 2.5% with a dose of 160 or less, 5.5% with a dose between 160 and 185, and 9.9% with a dose higher than 185). The incidence of severe urinary complications is also CT-dependent, with rates of 2% when the dose is less than 135 and 4% for when higher than 135.

Dose rate

In the randomised study by Patel et al [27] late rectosigmoid morbidity was significantly higher for the LDR patients: morbidity for grades 1-4 was 19.9% for LDR, but only 6.4% for HDR ($P = 0.001$). For severe complications, the difference was not significantly different ($P > 0.05$), but there was a trend in favour of HDR (2.4% LDR vs. 0.4% HDR). Although LDR is intrinsically less toxic to late-reacting tissues, the possible difference might be attributed to the more precise and controlled technique of source positioning during HDR (minutes of treatment) versus LDR (hours to days of treatment). However, there has been criticism of this study because the randomisation process was carried out by assigning alternating patients to each group.

In the overview by Fu [9], the average rates of moderate to severe complications were 12% for HDR and 18% for LDR. For the HDR treatments, the majority of the facilities employed Point A doses of 7-8 Gy/fraction for 3-6 fractions.

In the meta-analysis performed by Orton [25], complication rates were significantly lower for HDR. Severe complications were recorded in 2.2% of HDR patients and 5.3% of LDR patients. Although this study was not a randomised trial, statistical analysis of the data determined that the difference was significant ($P < 0.001$). One further item of interest from this study was the observation that complication rates for the HDR patients appeared to be related to the dose/fraction to Point A: both severe and moderate-plus-severe complication rates were statistically higher for patients treated with a dose/fraction > 7.5 Gy as compared to < 7.5 Gy.

Influence of the brachytherapy technique

Paris [26] compared the incidence of complications in 298 patients treated for cervical cancer as a function of the use of either a standard applicator of the Fletcher-Suit type or of minicolpostats with or without protection. In this series, grades 3 and 4 complications were found in 7.6% of the patients treated with the standard system, 26.9 % with the system using mini-ovoids and 36.6% with the system using mini-ovoids with protection ($P = 0.0006$). The exact aetiology of these complications could not be precisely determined. Crook [6] found rates of severe complications to be 29.5% and moderate complications to be 26% when the technique included a uterine catheter and vaginal cylinders, as compared to the technique using the standard Fletcher-Suit applicator ($P < 0.000001$). The brachytherapy technique alone can be responsible for complications.

Complications of combined radiotherapy and surgery

■ Surgery after radical radiation

In the literature, it is common to find rates of severe complications after combined radiotherapy and surgery on the order of 15% to 20% [5, 23, 31]. These high rates may be explained by the high pre-operative irradiation dose and the surgical indications, which are reserved for barrel-shaped tumours which are often bulky.

Mendenhall [23] reported on 150 patients with stage Ib et IIa-b cervical cancers larger than 6 cm. The risk of complications requiring hospitalisation was 16% in 75 patients treated with extrafascial hysterectomy after irradiation, a hysterectomy after radical EBRT and BT radiotherapy, as compared to 5% after radical radiotherapy. The same has been reported by others, who found higher fistulisation rates in patients treated with radiotherapy followed by extrafascial hysterectomy [7].

■ Tailored preoperative brachytherapy and surgery

In a series of 441 patients, Gerbaulet [11] used the Franco-Italian glossary [4] and reported complication rates of 44% for grade 1, 27% for grade 2 and 4.7% for grades 3 or 4.

These complication rates are particularly low. Calais [3] reported a complication rate for grade 3 of 6% in 115 patients treated by BT and surgery. These severe complications developed in 7 patients, of whom 4 had serious oedema of a lower limb.

In general, in the treatment of cervical cancer at early stages, combined brachytherapy and surgery gives excellent results in terms of both local control and the rate of complications. Decreasing the complication rates requires adaptation of the brachytherapy to the surgery (and vice versa), as well as a better knowledge of the limitations concerning doses to critical organs, according to the recommendations of the ICRU [17].

Chemoradiation

Both radiotherapy and chemotherapy are potentially toxic treatments and the combination of modalities may lead to added acute and late morbidity. The addition of chemotherapy is generally associated with more haematological and acute gastro-intestinal side effects than after radiotherapy alone. However, these acute side effects are usually transient and self-limiting or can be resolved with medical management. The regimen with CDDP weekly seems to be less toxic than a combination with polychemotherapy. The incidence of grades 3 and 4 acute haematological toxicity is twice as high after combination Hydroxyurea-CDDP and RT than after weekly cisplatin and radiotherapy ($P < 0.001$) [34].

Late complications are much less well described in published randomised studies, due to the limited follow-up of the patients. There is no mention of the incidence of late complications in the GOG 120 trial [34]. The only information about the incidence of late effects in the report of GOG 123 [18] is the statement that "very few patients required surgical intervention for obstruction or formation of a fistula and these patients were equally divided between the two groups."

Late complications are described in detail only in RTOG trial 9001 [24]. In the radiotherapy only arm, 10% of patients developed grade 4 complications (irreversible functional damage necessitating major therapeutic intervention) and 1% developed grade 3 damage (severe symptoms which had a significant negative impact on daily activities). The incidence of severe complications was similar in the chemoradiation group: 8% grade 4 and 4% grade 3 damage. The rather high incidence of severe late effects may be related to the high radiation doses given (at least 85 Gy to point A).

Fractionating and the type of brachytherapy used may be important in avoiding an increased incidence of complications following combined therapy. In all 3 studies published in full, external beam radiotherapy was given using ±10% lower total doses (45 Gy instead of 50 Gy) and smaller daily fraction sizes (1.8 Gy instead of 2 Gy) to avoid late toxicity. Brachytherapy was carried out using low dose rate (LDR) brachytherapy.

Deviation from this fractionation schedule can lead to serious problems. High dose rate brachytherapy (30 Gy in 3 weekly fractions) was associated with a 28% incidence of severe gastrointestinal complications in a phase I/II study of weekly cisplatin (30 mg/m^2) and external beam radiotherapy (46 Gy in 2 Gy fractions). Similarly, a study of 29 patients treated by hyperfractionated radiotherapy (1.2 Gy twice daily) and 3 weekly cisplatin plus fluorouracil had an unacceptably high incidence of severe late effects (21% grade 3, 28% grade 4).

Conclusions

Radiotherapy is feasible and effective in almost all patients with early cervical cancer.

Survival rates and local control results obtained by radical radiotherapy combining external beam irradiation with uterovaginal brachytherapy for stage I-II cervix cancer are similar to those obtained by radical surgery. This has been demonstrated in large retrospective series [16, 25, 29], as well as in a randomised trial on stage I-IIa cervical cancer [21]. In this randomised trial, grade 2-3 complications requiring medical or surgical treatment occurred in 12% of the radical radiation arm, versus 28% of the surgery group. However, complications were not significantly different in the surgery only subgroup (31%) as compared to the combined surgery and radiotherapy subgroup (27%). It seems that radiation limited to the pelvis does not significantly increase complication rates after surgery and that the latter may be more important.

Optimal results in radical radiotherapy can be obtained by defining the target volume and the critical organs with sectional imaging and adapting dose distribution to the individual variations in patients. It is also mandatory to respect short overall treatment times (less than 55 days) to counteract tumour cell repopulation. Special attention should be paid to integrate brachytherapy into a narrow time schedule with external beam RT.

There are data that treating patients having a low haemoglobin level has a negative effect on outcome. Keeping Hb levels during treatment above 12 g is therefore strongly advised.

Recent data from randomised trials [18, 24, 34, 39] have shown a survival and local control benefit over radiotherapy alone.

However, it is not settled yet whether optimal radiotherapy with a short overall treatment is able to produce the same results, or whether it can be further improved by concomitant chemotherapy.

Complication rates after modern radical radiotherapy are low, in the order of 5-7% for stage I, and 9-12% for stage II. In a randomised trial [21] they are significantly lower (12% grades 2-3) than after radical surgery or a combination of surgery and postoperative pelvic radiotherapy (28%) (P = 0.0004). Urological complications especially are more frequent in operated patients.

These findings have to be considered when selecting patients with stage I-II cervical cancer for treatment. The choice will depend on the institute's protocol, the competence of the surgical and radiation staff, and the patient's age, menopausal status, general health status and tumour size, to obtain the best cure rates with the least complications. Certainly those patients with high risk factors for pelvic node involvement or positive section margins, such as patients with large tumour size or stage II, or proven pelvic node involvement at staging laparotomy, are good candidates for radical radiation treatment.

When radiotherapy is performed, special attention must be paid to respecting the radiobiological consequences of dose rate and fraction sizes, and the combination with chemotherapy.

The use of sectional imaging in external beam radiation, and recently also in brachytherapy, will certainly further improve the results of radiotherapy by improved coverage of the target volume and better sparing of normal tissues.

References

[1] Barillot I, Horiot JC, Maingon P, Truc G, Chaplin G, Comte J et al. Impact on treatment outcome and late effects of customised treatment planning in cervix carcinomas. Baseline results to compare new strategies. *Int J Radiat Oncol Biol Phys* 2000 ; 48 : 189-200

[2] Bush RS, Jenkin RD, Allt WE, Beale FA, Bean H, Dembo AJ et al. Definitive evidence for hypoxic cells influencing cure in cancer therapy. *Br J Cancer* 1978 ; 37 : 302-306

[3] Calais G, Le Floch O, Chauvet B, Raynaud-Bougnoux A. Carcinoma of the uterine cervix stage Ib and early stage II. Prognostic value of histological tumor regression after initial brachytherapy. *Int J Radiat Oncol Biol Phys* 1989 ; 17 : 1231-1235

[4] Chassagne D, Sismondi P, Horiot JC, Sinistrero G, Bey P, Zola P et al. A glossary for reporting complications of treatment in gynecological cancers. *Radiother Oncol* 1993 ; 26 : 195-202

[5] Coleman DL, Gallup DG, Wolcott HD, Otken LB, Stock RJ. Patterns of failure of bulky-barrel carcinomas of the cervix. *Am J Obstet Gynecol* 1992 ; 166 : 916-920

[6] Crook J, Esche B, Chaplain G, Isturiz J, Sentenac I, Horiot JC. Dose-volume analysis and the prevention of radiation sequelae in cervical cancer. *Radiother Oncol* 1987 ; 8 : 321-332

[7] Eifel P, Levenback C, Wharton J, Oswald MJ. Time course and incidence of late complications in patients treated with radiation therapy for FIGO stade Ib carcinoma of the uterine cervix. *Int J Radiat Oncol Biol Phys* 1995 ; 32 : 1289-1300

[8] FIGO. Annual report on the results of treatment in gynaecological cancer. *J Epidemiol Biostat* 1998 ; 23 : 20-26

[9] Fu KK, Phillips TL. High-dose rate vs low-dose rate intracavitary brachytherapy for carcinoma of the cervix. *Int J Radiat Oncol Biol Phys* 1990 ; 19 : 791-796

[10] Fyles AW, Milosevic M, Wong R, Kavanagh MC, Pintilie M, Sun A et al. Oxygenation predicts radiation response and survival in patients with cervix cancer. *Radiother Oncol* 1998 ; 48 : 149-156

[11] Gerbaulet A, Kunkler IH, Ker GR, Haie C, Michel G, Prade M et al. Combined radiotherapy and surgery: local control and complications in early carcinoma of the uterine cervix - the Villejuif experience 1975-1984. *Radiother Oncol* 1992 ; 23 : 66-73

[12] Gerstner N, Wachter S, Knocke TH, Fellner C, Wambersie A, Potter R. The benefit of Beam's Eye View based 3D treatment planning for cervical cancer. *Radiother Oncol* 1999 ; 51 : 71-78

[13] Girinski T, Péjovic-Lenfant MH, Bourhis J, Campana F, Cosset JM, Petit C et al. Prognostic value of hemoglobin concentrations and blood transfusions in advanced carcinoma of the cervix treated by RT: results of a retrospective study of 386 patients. *Int J Radiat Oncol Biol Phys* 1989 ; 16 : 37-42

[14] Girinski T, Rey A, Roche B, Haie C, Gerbaulet A, Randrianarivello H. Overall treatment time in advanced cervical carcinomas: a critical parameter in treatment outcome. *Int J Radiat Oncol Biol Phys* 1993 ; 27 : 1051-1056

[15] Haie-Meder C, Kramar A, Lambin P, Lancar R, Scalliet P, Bouzy J et al. Analysis of complications in a prospective randomized trial comparing two brachytherapy low dose rates in cervical carcinoma. *Int J Radiat Oncol Biol Phys* 1994 ; 29 : 953-960

[16] Horiot JC, Pigneux J, Pourquier H, Schraub S, Achille E, Keiling R et al. Radiotherapy alone in carcinoma of intact uterine cervix according to Fletcher guidelines: a French cooperative study of 1383 cases. *Int J Radiat Oncol Biol Phys* 1988 ; 14 : 605-611

[17] ICRU (International Commission on Radiation Units and Measurements). Dose and volume specification for reporting intracavitary therapy in gynecology, Report 38, Bethesda, 1985

[18] Keys HM, Bundy BN, Stehman FB, Muderspach LI, Chafe WE, Suggs CL et al. Cisplatin, radiation, and adjuvant hysterectomy compared with radiation and adjuvant hysterectomy for bulky stage IB cervical carcinoma. *N Engl J Med* 1999 ; 340 : 1154-1161

[19] Lancar R, Kramar A, Haie-Meder C, Lambin P, Bouzy J, Scalliet P et al. Méthode d'évaluation des complications tardives. Étude basée sur un essai de phase III comparant deux faibles débits de dose en curiethérapie gynécologique. *Bull Cancer* 1994 ; 81 : 632-637

[20] Lanciano RM, Won M, Coia LR, Hanks GE. Pretreatment and treatment factors associated with improved outcome in squamous cell carcinoma of the uterine cervix: a final report of the 1973 and 1978 Patterns of Care Study. *Int J Radiat Oncol Biol Phys* 1991 ; 20 : 667-676

[21] Landoni F, Maneo A, Colombo A, Placa F, Milani R, Perigo P et al. Randomised study of radical surgery versus radiotherapy for stage IB-IIA cervical cancer. *Lancet* 1997 ; 350 : 535-540

[22] Lowrey GC, Mendenhall WM, Million RR. Stage IB or IIA-B carcinoma of the intact uterine cervix treated with irradiation: a multivariate analysis. *Int J Radiat Oncol Biol Phys* 1992 ; 24 : 205-210

[23] Mendenhall WM, McCarty P, Morgan LS, Chafe WE, Million RR. Stage IB or IIa-b carcinoma of the intact uterine cervix > 6 cm in diameter: Is adjuvant extrafacial hysterectomy beneficial? *Int J Radiat Oncol Biol Phys* 1991 ; 21 : 899-904

[24] Morris M, Eifel P, Lu J, Grigsby PW, Levenback C, Stevens RE et al. Pelvic radiation with concurrent chemotherapy compared with pelvic and para-aortic radiation for high-risk cervical cancer. *N Engl J Med* 1999 ; 340 : 1137-1143

[25] Orton CG, Seyedsadr M, Somnay A. Comparison of high and low dose rate remote afterloading for cervix cancer and the importance of fractionation. *Int J Radiat Oncol Biol Phys* 1991 ; 21 : 1425-1434

[26] Paris KJ, Spanos WJ, Day TG, Jox B, Lindberg RD. Incidence of complications with minivaginal colpostats in carcinoma of the uterine cervix. *Int J Radiat Oncol Biol Phys* 1991 ; 21 : 911-917

[27] Patel FD, Sharma SC, Negi PS, Ghoshal S, Gupta BD. Low dose rate vs HDR brachytherapy in the treatment of carcinoma of the uterine cervix: a clinical trial. *Int J Radiat Oncol Biol Phys* 1994 ; 28 : 335-341

[28] Perez C, Breaux S, Bedwinck JM, Madoc-Jones H, Camel HM, Lurdy JA et al. Radiation therapy alone in the treatment of carcinoma of the uterine cervix II. Analysis of complications. *Cancer* 1984 ; 54 : 235-246

[29] Perez C, Fox S, Lockett MA, Grigsby PW, Camel HM, Galakatos A et al. Impact of dose in outcome of irradiation alone in carcinoma of the uterine cervix: analysis of two different methods. *Int J Radiat Oncol Biol Phys* 1991 ; 21 : 885-898

[30] Perez CA, Grigsby PW, Castro-Vita H, Lockett MA. Carcinoma of the uterine cervix. I. Impact of prolongation of overall treatment time and timing of brachytherapy on outcome of radiation therapy. *Int J Radiat Oncol Biol Phys* 1995 ; 32 : 1275-1288

[31] Perez CA, Kao MS. Radiation therapy alone or combined with surgery in the treatment of barrel-shaped carcinoma of the uterine cervix (stages Ib, IIa, IIb). *Int J Radiat Oncol Biol Phys* 1985 ; 11 : 1903-1909

[32] Petereit DG, Sarkaria JN, Chappell R, Fowler JF, Hartmann TJ, Kinsella TJ et al. Adverse effect of treatment prolongation in cervical carcinoma. *Int J Radiat Oncol Biol Phys* 1995 ; 32 : 1301-1307

[33] Rader JS, Haraf DJ, Halpern HJ, Rotmensch J, Spelbring DR, Sutton H et al. Radiation therapy in the treatment of cervical cancer: the University of Chicago/Michael Reese Hospital experience. *J Surg Oncol* 1990 ; 44 : 157-165

[34] Rose PG, Bundy BN, Watkins EB, Thigpen JT, Deppe G, Maiman MA et al. Concurrent cisplatin-based radiotherapy and chemotherapy for locally advanced cervical cancer. *N Engl J Med* 1999 ; 340 : 1144-1153

[35] Russel AH, Walter JP, Anderson MW, Zukkowski CL. Sagittal magnetic resonance imaging in the design of lateral radiation treatment protocols for patients with locally advanced squamous cancer of the cervix. *Int J Radiat Oncol Biol Phys* 1992 ; 23 : 449-455

[36] Shigematsu Y, Nishiyama K, Masaki N, Inoue T, Miyata Y, Ikeda H et al. Treatment of carcinoma of the uterine cervix by remotely controlled afterloading intracavitary radiotherapy with HDR: a comparative study with a low-dose rate system. *Int J Radiat Oncol Biol Phys* 1983 ; 9 : 351-356

[37] Sinistrero G, Sismondi P, Rumore A, Zola P. Analysis of complications of cervix carcinoma treated by radiotherapy using the Franco-Italian glossary. *Radiother Oncol* 1993 ; 26 : 203-221

[38] Sismondi P, Sinistrero G, Zola P, Volpe T, Ferraris R, Castelli GL et al. Complications of uterine cervix carcinoma treatments: the problem of a uniform classification. *Radiother Oncol* 1989 ; 14 : 9-17

[39] Whitney CW, Sause W, Bundy BN, Malfetano JH, Hannigan EV, Fowler WC et al. Randomized comparison of fluorouracil plus cisplatin versus hydroxyurea as an adjunct to radiation therapy in stages IIB-IVA carcinoma of the cervix with negative para-aortic lymph nodes. A SWOG study. *J Clin Oncol* 1999 ; 17 : 1339-1348

Chapter 9

Radiotherapy and surgical treatment of cervical carcinoma stages IB and II

Gilles Body, Anna-Maria Alonso, Fatoumata Diallo-Diabaté, Franck Perrotin, Philippe Bougnoux, Jacques Lansac, Olivier Le Floch

G Body, Professeur des Universités, Praticien Hospitalier, Service de Gynécologie Obstétrique C, Hôpital Bretonneau, 2 Boulevard Tonnellé, 37044 Tours Cedex, France.

M Alonso, Interne de Spécialité, Service de Gynécologie Obstétrique C, Hôpital Bretonneau, 2, Boulevard Tonnellé, 37944 Tours Cedex, France.

F Diallo-Diabaté, Maître Assistante, Service de Gynécologie Obstétrique, Hôpital National du Point G, Bamako, Mali.

F Perrotin, Praticien hospitalier, Service de Gynécologie Obstétrique C, Hôpital Bretonneau, 2 boulevard Tonnellé, 37044 Tours Cedex, France.

P Bougnoux, Professeur des Universités, Praticien Hospitalien, Clinique d'Oncologie et Radiothérapie (CORAD), 2 boulevard Tonnellé, 37044 Tours Cedex, France.

J Lansac, Professeur des Universités, Praticien Hospitalier, Service de Gynécologie Obstétrique B, Hôpital Bretonneau, 2 boulevard Tonnellé, 37044 Tours Cedex, France.

O Le Floch, Professeur des Universités, Praticien Hospitalier, Clinique d'Oncologie et Radiothérapie (CORAD), Hôpital Bretonneau, 2 boulevard Tonnellé, 37044 Tours Cedex, France.

Radiotherapy and surgical treatment of cervical carcinoma stages IB and II

G Body, AM Alonso, F Diallo-Diabaté, F Perrotin, P Bougnoux, J Lansac, O Le Floch

Abstract. — *Combined radiation therapy and surgery is one of the reference treatments for stage IB and II cervical cancers.*

Treatment is based on the classical combination of uterovaginal curietherapy followed by vaginal hysterectomy with lymphadenectomy and, in certain cases, transcutaneous irradiation. In combined radiotherapy-surgery, the irradiation doses are lower and the surgery more limited than when either of these treatments is used alone. The goal of radiation therapy is to reduce, or in certain cases to sterilise, the cervical tumour. The goal of surgery is to remove the uterus, a potential source of recurrence, and the non-sterilised foci. Lymphadenectomy allows evaluation of the lymph node involvement, and when lymph nodes are involved, it orients the additional external radiation therapy required.

By means of a modulated combination of these two therapies, treatment is aimed at increasing the level of local control while reducing the risk of serious complications. The survival rates at 5 years are comparable to those after surgery or radiation therapy alone (> 90% when there is no lymph node involvement; between 55% and 70% when lymph nodes are involved).

Keywords: cervical carcinoma, surgery, radiotherapy.

Introduction

Combined radiation therapy and surgery (CRS) is one of the "conventional" therapeutic options in treating cervical carcinoma, as are surgery or radiation therapy alone, whereas treatment involving the use of laparoscopy represents a "modern" option.

CRS is used for cervical cancers of the following stages (according to the FIGO nomenclature: Montreal, 1998):

– IB: clinically visible lesions limited to the cervix uteri or preclinical cancers greater than stage IA (IB1: clinically visible lesions < 4.0 cm; IB2: clinically visible lesions > 4.0 cm).

– IIA: cervical carcinoma extended beyond the uterus, but not to the pelvic wall or to the lower third of the vagina, with no obvious parametrial involvement.

The treatment of cervical carcinoma stages IB and IIA (barrel-shaped excluded) is still controversial. The debate about whether to use either surgery or radiotherapy alone or radiotherapy associated with surgery has not been solved by a well-designed randomised prospective study. Data from the "Annual Report on the Results of Treatment in Gynaecological Cancer 1998" (published in the Journal of Epidemiology and Biostatistics, 1998) *(table I)* show that a minority of cervical carcinomas are treated by radiotherapy associated with surgery; however, these data are not exhaustive and are based on voluntary declarations.

Treatment by CRS is based on the conventional combination of uterovaginal curietherapy followed by vaginal hysterectomy with lymphadenectomy and, in some cases, transcutaneous irradiation. When CRS is used, the radiation doses are smaller and the surgery more limited than when either of these treatments is used alone. Thus:

– The aim of radiation therapy is to reduce, and even in a certain number of cases to sterilise, the cervical tumour; this reduces the extent of the surgical resection. In addition, curietherapy may be undertaken under better dosimetric conditions if the uterus is still in situ, thus improving local control.

– The aim of surgery is to remove the uterus, the potential source of recurrence, and the non-sterilised foci; this makes it possible to prevent risks of pyometra due to cervical stenosis and endometrial cancer following irradiation. Lymphadenectomy enables determination of the lymph node involvement, the prognostic value of which determines the supplementary external radiation therapy (required only for those women with lymph node involvement).

By means of a modulated combination of these two therapies, the aim of treatment is to increase the level of local control while reducing the risk of serious complications.

CRS is presented in this section on the basis of our experience, which is compared with data from the literature.

Table I. Cervical carcinoma stage IB and IIA. Patients treated in 1990-92. Distribution by stage and treatment. (Annual Report on the Results of Treatment in Gynaecological Cancer 1998)

Treatment	Stage IB	Stage IIa	Total
Surgery	1287 (44%)	73 (12.7%)	1360 (38.9%)
Radiotherapy	1194 (41%)	422 (73.3%)	1616 (46.2%)
Radiotherapy + Surgery	440 (15%)	80 (14%)	520 (14.9%)
Total	2921 (100%)	575 (100%)	3496 (100%)

Staging and classification

In our institution for the past 25 years, every patient with a biopsy-proven invasive cervical carcinoma has had a clinical evaluation – under general anaesthesia – performed jointly by the surgical gynaecologist and the radiation oncologist. These patients had previously undergone blood tests, including blood count with haemoglobin level, urea, creatinemia and electrolytes. Chest X-rays, an IVP and a lymphangiogram were included in the staging program. More recently, CT scans and/or MRI have been added in selected cases. Cystoscopy was performed during the general anaesthesia. A cervico-vaginal print using Zelgan® paste was made in order to measure exactly the cervical size and vaginal lesions and to look for minimal vaginal extension.

Following this evaluation, a diagram of the lesion was drawn up, and the classification was established using the modified FIGO staging system, where stage II is divided into proximal stage II (IIp: involvement of the upper third of the vagina and/or internal third of the parametrium) and distal stage II (IId: upper two-thirds of the vagina and/or internal two-thirds of the parametrium) as described in the Gustave Roussy Institute classification [10]. The treatment was defined and planned jointly at that time. Our general treatment policy was surgery alone for stage IA, radiotherapy alone for stages IId and III, and associated radiation and surgery for central pelvic tumours stages IB and IIp.

Techniques

▪ Surgery

In CRS, surgery is based on vaginal hysterectomy with lymphadenectomy. In contrast to surgery alone, the surgical excision is more limited, particularly in the dissection of the ureters and the parametria. Pelvic lymphadenectomy, by contrast, is the same as for surgery alone: it involves complete lymph node dissection involving the primary external and internal iliac chains.

Two major types of resection of the genital apparatus are used:

– Extrafascial hysterectomy in which the cardinal ligaments are sectioned level with the genital apparatus. The ureter is not uncrossed and the vagina is sectioned just below (no more than 1 cm) its insertion in the cervix.

– Proximal or "modified" radical vaginal hysterectomy: the cardinal ligaments are sectioned at a slight distance from the genital apparatus, directly in line with the ureter, inside the external pillar of the bladder. The vascularisation of the ureter is to a large extent preserved by a limited dissection: its connections with the peritoneum are preserved and, lower down, the dissection is continued on the internal aspect of the ureter, its intraligamental and preligamental portions being reflected forwards and outwards. The paracolpium is then sectioned in such a way that it is possible to remove a vaginal collar of at least 3 cm. If the carcinoma is extended into the vagina, the excision must be continue some distance beyond the lesions (one, or preferably two, centimetres).

As concerns the adnexa, where preservation is sought the ovaries may be transposed some distance from the radiation fields to the parietocolonic fossae, where they are fixed and identified by clips pedunculated on the lumbo-ovarian pedicles.

- ## Radiation therapy

Intracavitary radiotherapy (ICRT)

When the first treatment was brachytherapy, it was usually performed at the time of initial evaluation under general anaesthesia. A vesical tube was introduced into the bladder and the balloon filled with 7 cm^3 of iodine fluid in order to visualise the trigone position. Most of the time (85%), we used an individual vaginal mould prepared for each patient according to the Chassagne and Pierquin technique [10]. In a few cases, the Fletcher-Suit vaginal applicator was used. However, a rigid curved metal Fletcher uterine applicator was used in order to maintain the uterus in an anteverted position during the application to avoid excessive irradiation of the rectum. This applicator was introduced as far as the uterine fundus.

Dummy run lead sources were introduced into the uterine and vaginal tubes. The length of the uterine source was between 50 and 85 mm in order to have 10 to 15 mm projecting into the vagina. The length of the two vaginal sources was between 24 and 36 mm depending on the size of the vagina.

Antero-posterior and lateral X-ray films were taken to confirm the correct position of the applicator and to contribute to dosimetry.

Computerised dosimetry was carried out according to Report 38 by the ICRU (International Commission on Radiation Units and Measurements). The dose per day was calculated to several specific normal tissue reference points (bladder, rectum, vagina) as well as to the pelvic lymph nodes. Isodose curves were drawn in three planes (frontal, sagittal and "lymphatic trapezoid").

The duration of treatment was determined on an individual basis. Because the aim of the brachytherapy in this radiosurgical approach was not to destroy a macroscopic tumour but rather to sterilise a microscopic lesion, the dose delivered to the normal tissue was the main parameter in calculating the duration of irradiation. The dose to the bladder and to the rectal reference points did not exceed 65 Gy and the dose to the vaginal surface was not greater than 120 Gy. However, the 60 Gy isodose curve should include the tumour, the cervix and the proximal parametrium in order to deliver a microscopic tumoricidal dose to this clinical target volume.

In patients having a small tumour and excellent vaginal anatomy, it was easy to deliver a high dose to the target volume with a very low risk of complications. On the contrary, patients having a large tumour or a narrow vagina were not good candidates for initial intracavitary irradiation. In this case, external beam radiotherapy should be added to reduce the tumour volume prior to brachytherapy.

Following dosimetry, intracavitary therapy was started by remote after-loading with a Curietron. Cesium 137 sources were used with an activity necessary to deliver a dose rate of 0.50 to 0.60 Gy/h of the 60 Gy reference isodose, which is in a low dose range. Most of the patients were treated with only one application. Therefore, for patients who had brachytherapy alone before surgery, the time to deliver the 60 Gy of the reference isodose was around 120 hours (5 days). For patients who received external irradiation prior to brachytherapy, the duration of intracavitary irradiation was shorter and in relation to the external beam irradiation dose.

According to ICRU Report no. 38, doses were specified in terms of:

– a description of the reference volume encompassed by the 60 Gy isodose, including the height (H), width (W) and thickness (T).

– calculated values of the dose to specific normal tissue reference points within the treatment volume (bladder, rectum, vagina, pelvic lymph nodes). All these parameters were recording in a data base.

External beam radiotherapy (EBRT)

When indicated, EBRT was delivered using high energy photon beams, initially with a cobalt unit and since 1981 with a 25 MV Linac®. Patients were treated 5 times a week with a fraction of 1.8 to 2 Gy per day. The treatment technique and cerubend blocking were carefully tailored to encompass the patient's known disease and the potential sites of microscopic disease. In the anterior and posterior fields, the lower border was generally placed at mid-pubis and the upper border at the L4-L5 space unless the para-aortic nodes were deemed at risk. Lateral borders included iliac nodes with a margin of 1 to 1.5 cm when they were visualised on the lymphangiogram, or at least 1 cm outside the pelvic margins. If lateral fields were used, the anterior border included the tip of the pubis and the posterior border, including the sacrum in order to irradiate the uterosacral and cardinal ligaments.

Post-operatively, EBRT was indicated when pathological nodes where found in the lymphadenectomy specimen. Then, a dose of 45 to 55 Gy was delivered through anterior (AP) and posterior (PA) fields with central pelvic shielding to protect the ICRT area. The area irradiated was usually limited to the pelvis unless there was common iliac node involvement, in which case the volume was extended to the para-aortic nodes.

Pre-intracavitary EBRT was used to shrink bulky endocervical or exocervical tumours (larger than 4 cm in diameter), so as to optimise the ICRT geometry. Initially, the total dose was limited to 20 Gy to the pelvis using AP-PA fields with no central shielding. Then ICRT was limited to an additional dose of 40 Gy of the reference isodose 60 Gy (20 + 40). In several patients with bulky central disease, we found pelvic node involvement, and we felt that delivering an additional dose limited to 35 Gy was not radiobiogically optimal, given the interval of more than 2 months between the two EBRT treatments. Then in 1981, when we were able to irradiate with 25 MV photons, we decided (when indicated), to use a higher dose to the pelvis (up to 45 to 55 Gy with central shielding at 45 Gy) and to treat the microscopic involvement of the nodes with irradiation so that the surgical approach was limited to colpohysterectomy without lymphadenectomy. Additional ICRT was limited to 15 Gy of the reference isodose, 60 Gy (45 + 15).

Advantages and disadvantages

Advantages

There are essentially three advantages:

– **The possibility of preserving the ovaries.** Preliminary radiotherapy causes systematic and definitive sterilisation, which can only be avoided by preliminary ovarian transposition and hence by preliminary surgery. Preservation may be justified by the lack of hormone dependency of cervical carcinoma and the exceptional nature of the ovarian metastases in well-selected indications. It can only be meaningful for younger women (under 35 years of age, maximum 40 years) with a small stage IB epidermoid carcinoma (cervical tumours of less than 2 cm) in the absence of vascular emboli and lymph node involvement.

– **Sterilisation of the cervix. T**he absence of a residual tumour or microscopic residual disease in the surgical specimen after irradiation constitutes a good prognostic factor [20, 22]. This concept was confirmed by our experience involving 119 patients with bulky stage IB or IIA cervical carcinomas treated by pre-operative radiotherapy; in 60% of the cases, sterilisation of the cervix was complete, in 10% a small residual tumour persisted, and in 30% a large residual tumour remained. Comparison of the residue-free group and the bulky residual tumour group showed that the five-year relapse-free survival rate was respectively 72% and 48% (statistically significant differences with $P < 0.0001$). In this study, as in others [9, 30], it was apparent that in a multivariate analysis the principal factor for radiosensitivity was the patient's haemoglobin level at the beginning of treatment (< 120 g/L or > 120 g/L) with five-year global survival rates of 18% and 45% ($P < 0.05$). The other factors were the FIGO stage, the histological type (a poorer response was observed in the case of adenocarcinoma) and the volume of the isodose 60.

– **External irradiation only in the case of lymph node involvement:** histological lymph node involvement is a key prognostic factor. This results in external irradiation being performed in only 8 to 23% of stage I and 30 to 37% of stage II cancers.

Disadvantages

These are based on:

1) The complications [3], which are related to the extent of the surgical resection and the experience of the surgeon, together with the doses used and the areas involved in the radiotherapy. CRS is a therapeutic option that yields comparable complication rates to those of the other methods, as long as there is very close collaboration between the surgical and radiotherapy teams, both of which must have considerable experience.

– **Operative mortality**: its frequency is low, not exceeding 1% in the great majority of literature series; it is non-existent (0/326) in our experience. The main causes of mortality are essentially thrombo-embolic complications, which are much more frequent than massive haemorrhagic complications or severe infections.

– **Urological complications**: the most serious are vesicovaginal or ureterovaginal fistulae: the overall rate in our experience is 2.7% (9/326). Ureteral stenoses responsible for ureterohydronephrosis are due to scar tissue formation enveloping the terminal ureter, which may be associated with extrinsic compression by a pelvic lymphocele or haematoma. Usually asymptomatic, they are detected by renal ultrasonography carried out in the third postoperative month. Finally, urodynamic studies show the frequency of abnormalities, which are also found after surgery or radiotherapy alone, in the form of vesical instability, residual urine and transmission defects [17].

– **Digestive complications**: rectovaginal fistulae are exceptional; in our experience, the rate is 1.2% (4/326).

– **Lymphoceles** are observed in 0.5% to 3.6% of cases. Apart from the cases that resolve spontaneously, they may require one or more evacuation punctures and, in exceptional cases surgical revision, essentially for bulky and generally compressive lymphoceles; in this type of situation, a digestive fistula involving fistulisation of the lymphocele into the ileum has even been reported [8]. Pelvic haematomas are slightly more frequent (2.5 to 7.5% of cases).

– **Lower limb lymphoedema** appears to be infrequent (< 5% of cases), but may be incapacitating when it becomes extensive or does not respond to physiotherapy. The incidence is possibly underestimated, to judge by a Scandinavian study [31] in which 28% of patients had a slight increase (> 5%), 6% a moderate increase (> 10%), 7% a severe increase (> 15%), and in 22% of the cases the lymphoedema was symptomatic.

– An **effect on sexuality** however is very common: 20 to 25% of patients have sexual dysfunction and 6 to 20% cease all sexual activity. This is due to the shortening of the vagina and to the post-radiotherapeutic vaginal and pelvic fibrosis, not to mention the psychological factors [7].

2) The difficulties of treating complications and correcting pelvic recurrences: in the case of a gastrointestinal or urinary fistula or stenosis, surgical treatment involves a high failure rate, often requiring the creation of permanent urinary or digestive shunts. The same applies in the case of a recurrence, where surgery usually represents the only resort.

3) There are a certain number of arguments against ovarian transposition: risk of ovarian dystrophy resulting in painful and enlarged cystic ovaries, sometimes requiring surgical revision [5]; risk of ovarian insufficiency after transposition; and obviously, risk of ovarian metastases to the transposed ovaries, which may occur even in cases where the prognosis is considered to be good [19].

Therapeutic indications

■ At the uterine level

The therapeutic indications are based essentially on the stage. The tumour size also has a major prognostic value, as has been found by the majority of authors [15], with a few exceptions such as Grigsby's study [12] in which tumour size had no effect on the prognosis in a group of patients all receiving pre-operative irradiation.

In the case of radiation therapy, the most recent literature confirms the results of older studies. External irradiation improves local control [27]; by contrast, its effect on survival is still being debated [13, 21, 28]. Since it also has its own morbidity, the indications must be carefully selected [29].

The role of chemotherapy, which is reserved for bulky and advanced tumours, will not be discussed here.

In our practice, apart from stage IB cervical carcinomas less than 1 cm which we treat initially by surgery alone, our indications may be summarised as follows:

– In the absence of medical contraindication, the association of radiotherapy and surgery is proposed to patients with a central pelvic tumour (stage IB1 > 1cm). Preoperative intracavitary brachytherapy follows six weeks later. Colpohysterectomy with iliac lymphadenectomy is the treatment of choice. No aortic node dissection is performed. Additional external iliac irradiation is done in cases of pelvic node involvement. In the event of primary iliac lymph node involvement, we undertake lumbo-aortic irradiation; however, extension of the radiation field to this region must be carefully weighed, as it is of limited value, particularly as it induces a certain degree of morbidity [25].

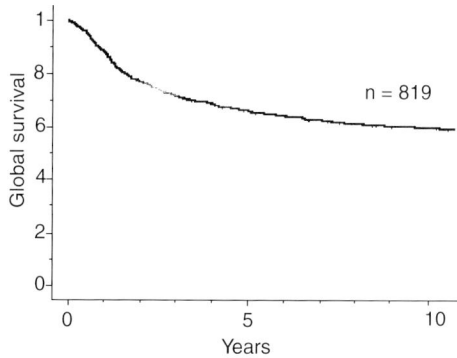

Figure 1. *Global survival curve for all cervical cancers (n=809), including 210 stage IB and 212 stage IIA.*

– In patients with a cervix diameter or tumour size larger than 4 cm, or where there is involvement of the central third of the vagina, initial intracavitary brachytherapy is not an appropriate technique due to the non-optimal and heterogeneous distribution of the dose. In this case, external pelvic irradiation up to 20 or 30 Gy is performed to reduce the size of the cervix and the tumour, followed by intracavitary application and the same surgery. However, because with large tumours the probability of involvement of pelvic nodes is higher, for this category of patients we decided to delivered a higher dose of external irradiation, up to 45 to 50 Gy, with a possible boost for the positive or doubtful nodes, followed by intracavitary irradiation and finally, adjuvant colpohysterectomy without lymphadenectomy. The aim of hysterectomy or adjuvant vaginal hysterectomy is to improve local (central pelvic) control of the disease: however this post-radiation surgery involves a higher rate of complications [18] and its value is the subject of controversy, leading some authors [14] to advise against it.

■ At the ovarian level

Apart from surgery alone and staging abdominal lymphadenectomy, there is no indication for ovarian transposition except in highly selected - and even then disputable - cases (young women with no risk factors for ovarian metastasis); under these circumstances, the vital prognosis is not affected [32]. Specific monitoring is required in all cases. To avoid an additional surgical procedure, ovarian transposition must be performed at the same time as the pre-operative uterovaginal curietherapy.

Results

The results from our experience are illustrated in figures *1* (global survival), *2* (global survival curve as a function of stage) and *3* (global survival as a function of stage and lymph node involvement).

The results in terms of survival are identical to those of the other treatments, surgery and radiation therapy alone; however, the comparisons are difficult. In particular, the randomised comparative [23] and non-comparative [24] studies of CRS and radiation therapy fail to show any difference in terms of local control, disease-free interval, global survival or complications. Tables *II*, *III* and *IV* show some results from literature.

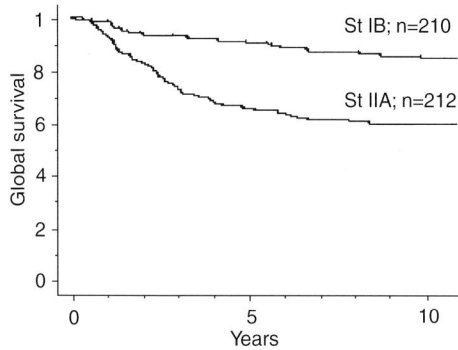

Figure 2. *Global survival curve for cervical cancer by stage.*

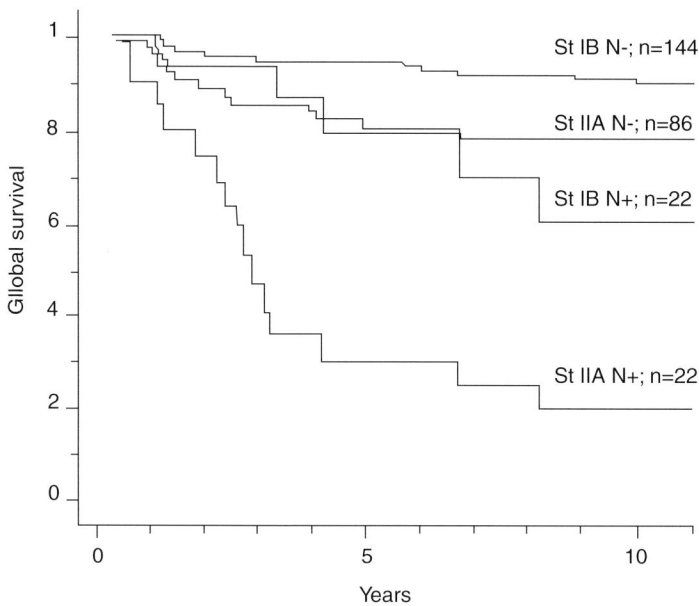

Figure 3. *Global survival curve for cervical cancer by stage and by lymph node involvement.*

The five-year survival rate in stages IB and IIA, all treatments combined, is 97.5 and 91.1%, respectively, in the absence of lymph node involvement, versus 65.9 and 55.0% in the case of lymph node involvement [2].

Conclusion

CSR is one of the three main therapeutic options for treatment of stage IB and IIA cervical carcinomas. The literature reveals no significant difference between these three methods, whether or not the tumour is less than four centimetres in size. For this reason, CSR remains one of the reference approaches to the treatment of cervical carcinoma.

Table II. Cervical carcinoma stage IB and IIA: results of the radio-surgical treatment.

Author	Number of Patients	Stage	Local control	Survival rate	Complications
Smales 1987 [26]	100	IB=74 pts IIA=8 pts	-	5 years * IB=85% IIA=100%	Grade III N-=5% N+=60%
Calais 1989 [4]	115	IB=70 pts IIA=45 pts	IB=100% IIA=93%	10 years ** IB=92% IIA=78%	Grade III 6%
Lasry 1998 [16]	415	T1=331 pts T2=84 pts	T1=93% T2=85%	10 years ** T1=82% T2=59%	Grade III 9.6%
Gerbaulet 1992 [11]	391	IB=288 pts IIA=103 pts	IB=92% IIA=89%	5 years * IB=88% IIA=87%	Grade III et IV=4.7%
Body, Lefloch 1997	461	IB=244 pts IIA=27 pts		IB=92.7 IIA=71.6	Grade III et IV=4.4%
Annual report 1998	520	IB=440 pts IIA=80 pts	-	5 years ** IB=83.6% IIA=80.3%	-

Pts : Patients
*Relapse free survival rate
** Overall survival rate

Table III. Cervical carcinoma stage IB and IIA: Comparison between radiotherapy and radio-surgical treatment.

Authors	Number of patients	Stage	Local control	Survival rate	Complications
Perez 1987 [23] Randomised	RT=56	IB+IIA	91%	5 years ** IB=89% IIA=56%	Grade III-IV 10%
	RT+surg=62		92%	IB=80% IIA=79%	8%
Bachaud 1991 [1] Non randomised	RT=139 Rt+surg=115	Ib+IIA+IIB	84% 87%	5 years ** 82% 82%	Grade III-IV 2% 6%
Pernot 1995 [24] Non randomised	IB RT=83 IIBRT=173 IB RT+surg=205 IIb RT+surg=19	IB+IIA	87% - 92% -	5 years ** 91% 68% 76% 57%	Grade III-IV 4.2% 3.3%

*Relapse free survival rate
** Overall survival rate

Table IV. Cervical carcinoma stage IB and IIA: comparison between radiotherapy and radio-surgical treatment. (Annual Report on the Results of Treatment in Gynaecological Cancer 1998). Non randomised study.

Treatment	Stage	Mean age	Number of patients	Overall surival rate at 5 years
Surgery alone	IB	44.8	1287	90.3%
	IIA	49.7	73	65.9%
Radiotherapy alone	IB	55.1	1194	72.2%
	IIA	59.7	422	64.6%
RT + surgery	IB	48.2	440	83.6%
	IIA	55.4	80	80.3%

References

[1] Bachaud JM, Fu RC, Delannes M. Non randomised comparative study of irradiation alone or in combination with surgery in stage IB, IIA and proximal IIB carcinoma of the cervix. *Radiother Oncol* 1991 ; 22 : 104-110

[2] Benedet J, Odicino F, Maisonneuve P et al. Carcinoma of the cervix uteri. *J Epidemiol Biostat* 1988 ; 3 : 5-34

[3] Body G, Calais G, Dargent G, Horiot JC, Lansac J, Le Floch O. Le traitement de cancer du col. *Encycl Méd Chir* (Éditions Scientifiques et Médicales Elsevier SAS, Paris), Gynécologie, 600-A-20, 600-A-30, 1990

[4] Calais G, Le Floch O, Chauvet B. Carcinoma of the uterine cervix stage IB and early stage II. Pronostic value of the histological tumor regression after initial brachytherapy. *Int J Radiat Oncol Biol Phys* 1989 ; 17 : 1231-1235

[5] Chambers SK, Chambers JT, Holm C, Peschel RE, Schwartz PE. Sequelae of lateral ovarian transposition in unirradiated cervical cancer patients. *Gynecol Oncol* 1990 ; 39 : 155-159

[6] Chassagne D, Sismondi D, Horiot JC. A glossary for reporting complications of treatment in gynaecological cancers. *Radiother Oncol* 1993 ; 26 : 195-202

[7] Flay LD, Matthews JH. The effects of radiotherapy and surgery on the sexual function of women treated for cervical cancer. *Int J Radiat Oncol Biol Phys* 1995 ; 31 : 399-404

[8] Fotiou SK, Tserkezoglou AJ, Steinhauer G, Papailiou J, Tavernarakis A. Pelvic lymphocysts after radical hysterectomy and lymphadenectomy. *Eur J Gynaecol Oncol* 1994 ; 15 : 449-454

[9] Fyles AW, Pintilie M, Kirkbride P, Levin W, Manchul LA, Rawlings GA. Prognostic factors in patients with cervix cancer treated by radiation therapy: result of a multiple regression analysis. *Radiother Oncol* 1995 ; 35 : 107-117

[10] Gerbaulet A, Michel G, Haie-Meder C, Castaigne D, Lartigau E, L'Homme C et al. The role of low dose rate brachytherapy in the treatment of cervix carcinoma: experience of the Gustave Roussy institute 0n 1245 patients. *Eur J Gynaecol Onol* 1995 ; 16 : 461-475

[11] Gerbaulet G, Kunkler IH, Kerr GR. Combined radiotherapy and surgery: local control and complications in early carcinoma of the uterine cervix: the Villejuif experience 1975-1984. *Radiother Oncol* 1992 ; 23 : 66-73

[12] Grigsby PW, Perez CA, Chao KS, Elbendary A, Herzog TJ, Rader JS, Mutch DG. Lack of effect of tumor size on the prognosis of carcinoma of the uterine cervix stage IB and IIA treated with preoperative irradiation and surgery. *Int J Radiat Oncol Biol Phys* 1999 ; 45 : 645-651

[13] Hopkins MP, Morley GW. Radical hysterectomy versus radiation therapy for stage IB squamous cell cancer of the cervix. *Cancer* 1991 ; 68 : 272-277

[14] Kim HK, Silver B, Berkowitz R, Howes A. Bulky, barrel-shaped cervical carcinoma (stages IB, IIA, IIB): the prognostic factors for pelvic control and treatment outcome. *Am J Clin Oncol* 1999 ; 22 : 232-236

[15] Lambin P, Kramar A, Haie-Meder C, Castaigne D, Scalliet P, Bouzy J et al. Tumour size in cancer of the cervix. *Acta Oncol* 1998 ; 37 : 729-734

[16] Lasry S, Cohen-Solal C, Hasene K. Long term results of radiosurgical treatment of operable carcinoma of the cervix uteri. *Bull Cancer* 1990 ; 77 : 355-362

[17] Lin HH, Sheu BC, Lo MC, Huang SC. Abnormal urodynamic findings after radical hysterectomy or pelvic irradiation for cervical cancer. *Int J Gynaecol Obstet* 1998 ; 63 : 169-174

[18] Mendenhall WM, McCarty PJ, Morgan LS, Chafe WE, Million R. Stage IB or IIA-B carcinoma of the intact uterine cervix greater than or equal to 6cm in diameter: is adjuvant extrafascial hysterectomy beneficial ? *Int J Radiat Oncol Biol Phys* 1991 ; 21 : 899-904

[19] Michel G, Zarca D, Guettier X, Castaigne D, Charpentier P. Une observation de métastase ovarienne sur ovaire transposé, après traitement radiochirurgical d'un épithélioma épidermoïde du col utérin. Comment minimiser le risque ? *Cah Cancer* 1989 ; 1 : 121-123

[20] Mundt AJ, Waggoner S, Herbst A, Rotmensch J. Preoperative intracavitary brachytherapy in early-stage cervical carcinoma. *Am J Clin Oncol* 1999 ; 22 : 73-77

[21] Okada M, Kigawa J, Minagawa Y, Kanamori Y, Shimada M, Takahashi M et al. Indication and efficacy of radiation therapy following radical surgery in patients with stage IB to IIB cervical cancer. *Gynecol Oncol* 1998 ; 70 : 61-64

[22] Paley PJ, Goff BA, Minudri R, Greer BE, Tamimi HK, Koh WJ. The prognostic significance of radiation dose and residual tumor in the treatment of barrel-shaped endophytic cervical carcinoma. *Gynecol Oncol* 2000 ; 76 : 373-379

[23] Perez CA, Camel HM, Kao MS, Hederman MA. Randomized study of preoperative radiation and surgery or irradiation alone in the treatment of stage IB and IIA carcinoma of the uterine cervix: final report. *Gynecol Oncol* 1987 ; 27 : 129-140

[24] Pernot M, Hoffstetter S, Peiffert D, Carolus JM, Guillemin F, Verhaeghe JL et al. Statistical study of a series of 672 cases of carcinoma of the uterine cervix. Results and complications according to age modalities of treatment. *Bull Cancer* 1995 ; 82 : 568-581

[25] Rotman M, Choi K, Guse C, Marcial V, Hornback N, John M et al. Prophylactic irradiation of the para-aortic lymph node chain in stage IIB and bulky stage IB carcinoma of the cervix, initial treatment results of RTOG 7920. *Int L Radiat Oncol Biol Phys* 1990 ; 19 : 513-521

[26] Smales E, Perry CM, Baker JW. The role of combined therapy in the management of stage one and two carcinoma of the cervix. *Eur J Gynaecol Oncol* 1987 ; 8 : 578-584

[27] Tsai CS, Lai CH, Wang CC, Chang JT, Chang TC, Tseng CJ et al. The prognostic factors for patients with early cervical cancer treated by radical hysterectomy and postoperative radiotherapy. *Gynecol Oncol* 1999 ; 75 : 328-333

[28] Uno T, Ito H, Itami J, Yasuda S, Isobe K, Hara R et al. Postoperative radiation therapy for stage IB-IIB carcinoma of the cervix with poor prognostic factors. *Anticancer Res* 2000 ; 20 : 2235-2239

[29] Vinod SK, MacLeod CA, Dalrymple C, Elliott P, Atkinson K, Carter J et al. Surgery and post-operative radiotherapy for early stage cervical cancer. *Aust N Z J Obstet Gynaecol* 2000 ; 40 : 66-69

[30] Werner-Wasik M, Schmid CH, Bornstein L, Ball HG, Smith DM, Madocjones H. Prognostic factor for local and distant recurrence in stage I and II cervical carcinoma. *Int J Radiat Oncol Biol Phys* 1995 ; 32 : 1309-1317

[31] Werngren-Elgstrom M, Lidman D. Lymphoedema of the lower extremities after surgery and radiotherapy for cancer of the cervix. *Scand J Plast Reconstr Surg Hand Surg* 1994 ; 28 : 289-293

[32] Windbichler GH, Müller-Holzner E, Nicolussi-Leck G, Meisel U, Dapunt O, Marth C. Ovarian preservation in the surgical treatment of cervical carcinoma. *Am J Obstet Gynecol* 1999 ; 180 : 963-969

Chapter 10

Laparoscopic approach: new concepts of treatment of cervical carcinoma stages I and II

Denis Querleu, Eric Leblanc

D Querleu, *Professeur de gynécologie-obstétrique.*
E Leblanc, *Chirurgien.*
Département de Cancérologie gynécologique, Centre Oscar Lambret, Lille, France.

Laparoscopic approach: new concepts
of treatment of cervical carcinoma stages I and II

D Querleu, E Leblanc

Abstract. — *Laparoscopic surgery has recently been introduced in the field of cervical cancer treatment. Like any surgery, it may be used as a staging procedure or as an approach to the surgical management of cervical cancer. Since the issue is still controversial, and the feasibility of randomised studies is extremely low, a careful prospective evaluation of cases is needed to make sure that the introduction of minimal access surgery, including laparoscopic and vaginal approaches, does not impair patient outcome.*

Keywords: cervical carcinoma, laparoscopic surgery, pelvic lymphadenectomy, radical hysterectomy.

Staging

Clinical staging of cervical carcinomas is still the mainstay of classification. Intravenous pyelography and cystoscopy are also routinely performed. None of these investigations evaluates lymph node status. Node involvement is, however, a major prognostic factor of cervical cancer. The sensitivity and specificity of imaging techniques (CT scan, ultrasound, MRI) in the detection of nodal involvement are unsatisfactory. Pathological examination is the only reliable method for appraising the status of lymph nodes. However, samples are usually taken either during a presurgical staging laparotomy, adding significant morbidity, or during surgical treatment, at a time when primary decisions about treatment have already been taken. The rationale for laparoscopic pelvic lymphadenectomy is to provide reliable information concerning the node status through a minimal access procedure.

■ General principles

Pelvic node involvement is the single most significant factor in the prognosis of early cervical carcinomas. The risk of "skip" metastases to the para-aortic area is negligible in patients with tumours smaller than 3 centimetres and negative pelvic nodes. As a consequence, stage IB-IIB cases with negative pathological staging may be cured by local therapy (brachytherapy alone or radical hysterectomy). On the other hand, radical hysterectomy does not seem justified when metastatic nodes are present, and in our institution, positive node patients are offered radiation therapy only. In addition, some stage IA2 or early invasive cervical carcinomas without pelvic node metastasis can be treated by radical trachelectomy, a fertility-sparing procedure [10].

The risk of para-aortic node involvement is significant in patients with locally advanced cervical carcinomas and pelvic nodal metastases. The latter may even occasionally be observed in the absence of positive pelvic nodes in patients with stage I and II large cervical tumours. Sampling of the para-aortic lymph nodes has been suggested as a means of identifying those patients with extra-pelvic spread in whom standard therapy involving pelvic surgery or radiation fields would consequently fail.

The risk/benefit assessment of surgical staging is a subject of debate. Potential perioperative and late complications as well as difficulties treating patients with para-aortic nodal metastases do not favour routine surgical staging. However, it is necessary in investigational settings to assess the para-aortic nodal status of high-risk patients in therapeutic trials involving para-aortic irradiation and/or systemic chemotherapy. A proportion of patients without metastatic para-aortic nodes in the presence of advanced pelvic tumours undergo unnecessary extended field irradiation with subsequent complications and questionable therapeutic value. The probability that extended field radiation without information on the para-aortic node status will improve therapy is likely to be no more than 4%, which justifies some sort of surgical staging.

In conclusion, an elective pelvic lymphadenectomy provides satisfactory staging in the majority of early (IA2 and IB1) cervical carcinomas. In addition, para-aortic lymphadenectomy may benefit patients with IB2-II cervical carcinomas and/or with pelvic node metastasis.

■ Technical considerations

Endoscopic techniques are described elsewhere [10] and will not be developed here. Pelvic node dissection for the staging of early cervical carcinomas may be limited to the lymphatics of the interiliac area (between the bifurcation of the branches of the common iliac arteries), including the obturator nodes and those located between the external and internal iliac arteries.

Extended dissection for staging advanced cervical carcinomas must include removal of the common iliac and para-aortic nodes. The surgical landmark for nodal dissection in cervical carcinomas is usually the origin of the inferior mesenteric artery, but recent data show that the aortic dissection should be extended to the level of the renal veins, particularly on the left side [9]. Section of ovarian arteries and of the right ovarian vein is not necessary, and only the identification of the left renal vein is required. The dissection is extended from the common iliac arteries up to the level of the left renal vein between the right and left ureters.

▪ Evolution of laparoscopic lymphadenectomy in cervical carcinomas

Minimal access surgery is better adapted to the concept of a staging procedure than laparotomy. Laparoscopy may offer the opportunity to assess nodal status before considering the extent of therapy.

In 1987, Dargent and Salvat described a panoramic, retroperitoneal approach for removal of the interiliac nodes [4]. In 1989 we described the technique of interiliac pelvic lymphadenectomy by laparoscopy [13]. Following earlier descriptions of para-aortic node samplings, or dissection of the lower two centimetres of the aorta, Childers et al described the first low elective para-aortic lymphadenectomies [1]. The same year (1991), we performed the first transperitoneal infrarenal para-aortic dissection [12]. Later, Dargent [3] developed an extraperitoneal endoscopic technique for aortic dissection which we have adopted [11].

These operations are not difficult for an experienced oncological surgeon and may be routinely carried out by laparoscopy. According to the experience of three of the leading teams in this field, the proportion of patients in whom the operation can be satisfactorily completed by this new approach is well over 90% [Childers, Querleu, Dargent, personal communications]. The goal of such a staging operation is to spare the negative node patient unnecessary pelvic or para-aortic irradiation, and the positive node patient unnecessary pelvic primary surgery or exenteration for pelvic recurrence.

▪ Results of laparoscopic pelvic lymphadenectomy in early cervical carcinomas

Laparoscopic pelvic lymphadenectomy appears to yield a satisfactory assessment of pelvic nodes with a minimum of surgical trauma. The number of nodes removed from the obturator area and medial chain of the external iliac nodes (averaging 20 in our current experience) is comparable to the number removed by laparotomy.

Dargent [2] reported 51 cases of cervical cancer managed with retroperitoneal lymphadenectomy and radical vaginal hysterectomy. The 3 year survival rate was 95.5% in negative node stage IB and IIA patients and 80% in negative node early IIB patients.

In our series, up to five years follow-up is available for 106 patients with early cervical carcinomas managed with laparoscopic pelvic lymphadenectomy. The quality of the pelvic dissection was checked by laparotomy in 68 patients. No residual positive nodes were found. At the time of writing, the four year life table survival rate is 83% for the entire group, and is similar to the survival of a historical group matched for age, stage and therapy [10]. All recurrences were observed in high-risk patients (young women with bulky tumours or adenocarcinoma). We observed three recurrences in the lateral pelvic area alone in 84 surgically treated, negative node patients. This 4% rate of purely lateropelvic recurrence, suggesting a growth of missed lymph nodes, is similar to the rate observed after laparotomy. The procedure is thus safe and accurate, and may be included in the staging and therapeutic strategy for cervical cancers.

In addition, it seems that the radiation therapy complication rate is lower after laparoscopic pelvic lymphadenectomy as compared to open staging. In a case control study of two groups of 26 patients with cervical cancer and positive pelvic nodes, we found a significantly lower grade 3-4 radiation therapy complication rate in the group of patients staged laparoscopically and submitted to radiation therapy only, as compared to patients managed by open radical surgery [10].

■ The new concept of parametrial lymphadenectomy

The removal of the parietal lymph nodes related to the uterus is generally referred to as "pelvic" lymphadenectomy. However, these nodes are not the only ones involved in the natural history of cervical carcinomas.

Some lymphatic channels are occasionally interrupted by one or (rarely) several nodes running along the uterine artery. They may be selectively removed by laparoscopy by blunt separation from the uterine artery, or their removal may be included in the removal of the entire uterine artery during radical hysterectomy. This step of the operation is quite feasible using laparoscopy as a part of a full laparoscopic hysterectomy, or preferably as part of a laparoscopically-assisted radical vaginal hysterectomy.

Much more frequently, lymph nodes are found in the cardinal ligament (named paracervix in the international anatomical classification). Girardi et al [5] found positive paracervical nodes in 22.5% of stage IB and II patients. They are anatomically spread, either in the proximal part of the ligament, close to the uterus, or in the distal part of the ligament, closer to the pelvic wall. Their involvement has a prognostic significance and their removal may reduce the rate of late lateropelvic recurrences. The proximal part of the ligament cannot be sampled without performing a radical hysterectomy, and cannot be included in a staging procedure. On the other hand, the cellulolymphatic component of the distal part of the ligament may be removed separately from the uterus and from the nerves and vessels of the cardinal ligament. We have labelled this dissection of the cardinal ligament "paracervical lymphadenectomy" and have described a laparoscopic technique for this operation [10].

Paracervical lymphadenectomy is not only a staging procedure, but may be considered as part of the surgical management of cervical carcinomas. Short-term fistula formation and long-term voiding difficulties are the two major adverse effects of radical hysterectomies. However, the complication rate is strikingly different according to the extent of removal of the cardinal ligament. It is quite low after "proximal" modified radical hysterectomy (type 2), and quite high after "distal" (type 3 or 4) radical hysterectomy. The fistula formation rate is as high as 5% to 10% compared to almost 0 after the "proximal" type of radical hysterectomy [8]. The long-term voiding difficulty rate may reach 40% after a "distal" operation, but is quite rare after a "proximal" one. Adding a parametrial lymphadenectomy to a proximal type radical hysterectomy leads to a de facto distal type of radical hysterectomy, while potentially dramatically reducing the complication rate.

In early clinical IB cervical cancers with small tumour volume (under 2 cm in maximum diameter or less than 10 cc in volume measured by MRI), the chance of involvement of the cardinal ligament is quite low, and a policy of proximal radical hysterectomy seems justified, showing less morbidity with comparable efficacy [7]. As a consequence, routine parametrial lymphadenectomy is not justified. However, the presence of diseased parietal lymph nodes is correlated with the presence of parametrial lymph nodes [5]. In the Girardi et al series, considering all cases of stage IB and II cervical cancers, the positivite rate for parametrial lymph nodes is 40% when parietal nodes are involved, compared to only 5% when the parietal nodes are negative. As a consequence, the logical strategy is to start the operation with a parietal pelvic lymphadenectomy. If the frozen section of the parietal dissection demonstrates positive nodes, a parametrial lymphadenectomy is indicated. In the same way, a cardinal ligament dissection may be necessary in cases with angiolymphatic space involvement.

In more advanced IB or IIA cervical cancers (2 to 4 cm or between 10 and 50 cc), the chances of involvement of the distal part of the cardinal ligament becomes significant. In the Girardi series, the positivity rate for parametrial nodes is 15%, 26% and 35%, respectively, when the tumour invades 40-60%, 60-80% or > 80% of the cervix. According to our policy, in such cases there is an elective indication for parametrial lymphadenectomy.

In cases of large tumour volume (more than 4 cm or 50 cc), we suggest primary external radiation therapy, and we do not perform interiliac lymphadenectomy as a staging procedure. As a consequence, we find no place for parametrial lymphadenectomy in these circumstances. Some other authors favour primary surgery. They may combine a laparoscopic parametrial lymphadenectomy and a classical abdominal radical hysterectomy, removing the entire uterine artery and the proximal part of the cardinal ligament by conventional means.

■ Results and rationale of extraperitoneal endoscopic aortic dissection in bulky or pelvic positive nodes for early stage cervical cancers

The results of this approach, which in our experience is adapted to the staging of bulky, early stage cervical cancers, are available in a series which also includes advanced cases [11]. However, the technical issues, complications and accuracy do not depend on the indication.

In this series, 53 patients underwent infrarenal aortic and common iliac dissection for the staging of bulky or advanced cervical carcinomas. The indication for extended nodal staging was bulky, early stage in 33 patients, FIGO stage III or distal IIb in 14 patients, non-bulky, early stage with microscopic, positive pelvic nodes in one patient and central recurrence in 5 patients. The node dissection template included the common iliac nodes, presacral, inframesenteric nodes, and the pre-aortic and lateroaortic infrarenal nodes. The operation was performed using endoscopic techniques with CO_2 insufflation of the extraperitoneal space. The procedure failed in 2 patients. Nine patients had node biopsy or selective removal of macroscopically positive nodes. In the 42 remaining patients, the average duration of the operation was 125.9 ± 31.8 minutes and the average number of nodes was 20.7. Overall, 17 patients had positive nodes, macroscopic in 9 patients, microscopic in 8; the positivity rate was 32%. Five complications occurred, four of them related to the extraperitoneal dissection technique. A peroperative complication occurred in one patient, in whom a lateral injury to a fixed and dilated ureter was managed by stenting. A postoperative complication occurred in another patient, in whom a retroperitoneal haematoma causing ileus and compression of the upper ureter was managed conservatively. Two symptomatic lymphocysts occurred, one of them requiring drainage under ultrasound guidance. All patients but one had external radiation therapy tailored according to the aortic node status. After an average follow-up of 12 months, 6 patients had persistent disease or it had recurred in the pelvic area, 8 in distant sites, and 2 in both pelvic and distant sites. The site of recurrence was distant or pelvic and distant in all positive node patients, and pelvic in all negative node patients but one. No patient recurred in the aortic or common area. Two patients suffered from radiation enteritis.

A significant proportion (11%) of patients with bulky tumours and 25% of patients with positive pelvic nodes have aortic metastasis. These figures are a clear rationale for assessment of the aortic nodes on a routine basis. Considering the complication rate and cost of a laparotomy for aortic lymphadenectomy, some investigators recently explored the feasibility of laparoscopic staging. It is not clear whether consequent complications of radiation therapy are actually reduced after extraperitoneal endosurgery, as compared to open extraperitoneal surgery. The complication rate of this purely diagnostic operation must be addressed and put into perspective with the complication rate of systematic, extended field radiation therapy, which is estimated to be in the range of 10%-14%. More precisely, the key issue is the additional complication rate of an extended field in randomised studies [6, 14] compared to a pelvic field which is estimated to be in the range of 4%.

In our series [11], two symptomatic lymphoceles and one ureteric injury were observed, for a complication rate of 5.7% (3/53), which does not differ from the complication rate observed in a series of open extraperitoneal lymph node dissection. If an additional case of incidental laparotomy is taken into account, the complication rate estimate is 7.6% (4/53). Only the latter complication required laparotomy and led to severe long-term side effects, for a grade 3 complication rate of 3%. This complication should no longer occur in the future as we now suture the fascia of the umbilical incision, and the grade 3 complication rate would have been zero if we had taken this precaution from the beginning. The severe complication rate of extraperitoneal endoscopic staging may thus prove to be extremely low, and to compare favourably with the additional complication rate related to extended field radiation therapy administered to all patients, regardless of their node status. In addition, a systematic dissection of the common iliac area may result in a reduction of the radiation field in negative node patients. The standard upper limit of the pelvic field is usually the junction of L4-L5. In our centre, the upper limit of the pelvic field will, in the future, be adapted to the radiological localisation of clips placed at the lower limit of the dissection during endosurgery, which is constantly below the level of the sacral promontory.

Surgical therapy

■ Concepts for surgical technique

When radical hysterectomy is required for cervical cancer, classical vaginal surgery may follow laparoscopic staging in the same session. Techniques of laparoscopic or laparoscopically-assisted radical hysterectomy have also been described. These techniques for radical cancer surgery are still investigational, but several teams have demonstrated their feasibility.

The term "radical" hysterectomy encompasses many different operations. We use only two terms, referring to two operations that are different in radicality. The only criterion we use is the extent of removal of the cardinal ligaments, given that the lateral extent is the main source of complications, including fistula formation and long-term voiding difficulties. "Proximal" or "modified" radical hysterectomy refers to those procedures in which only the proximal part of the parametria is excised medially to the level of the ureters, and corresponds to the Piver type 2. The uterosacral ligaments are also removed in their mid portion proximal to the uterus. The vagina is incised to leave a 2 cm margin. "Distal" or "classical" radical hysterectomy is the procedure which removes the entire parametria, as lateral as their insertion in the pelvic sidewall, and corresponds to the Piver type 3 or 4. The uterosacral ligaments are removed in toto. Again, the vagina is incised with a 2 cm margin.

Only the technique of modified radical hysterectomy will be addressed in this chapter. Proximal or modified radical hysterectomy (MRH) is indicated for early stage IB, less than 2 centimetres in diameter or not exceeding 10 cc, or after primary brachytherapy. In 1959, Mitra described a combination of abdominal and vaginal surgery in which pelvic lymphadenectomy and a section of the uterine vessels are performed abdominally using a retroperitoneal approach; the incision of the vagina and division of the cardinal ligaments are then performed vaginally. However, this technique implies two large inguinal incisions, and it is not clear whether it involves fewer complications than the standard abdominal approach. For all these reasons, the abdominal approach has remained the only widely accepted approach for the completion of modified radical hysterectomy and lymph node dissection.

The introduction of laparoscopic surgery in gynaecological oncology has had two consequences. First, it has elicited a revival of vaginal radical hysterectomy, giving birth to new variants of radical hysterectomy. Second, procedures similar to the standard surgery have been described, challenging the supremacy of abdominal surgery. The first historical application of panoramic endoscopic surgery in the field of gynaecological oncology was interiliac lymphadenectomy through a retroperitoneal approach. Daniel Dargent, the pioneer of this approach, had the idea of adding an endoscopic lymphadenectomy to a classical (distal) Schauta or a modified (proximal) Schauta operation. The goal was to overcome the lack of lymph node dissection in the vaginal procedure. The transumbilical approach was pioneered by our group. A few years later, leading teams in advanced laparoscopic surgery attempted radical operations using laparoscopic techniques. Later, we invented the idea that vaginal radical hysterectomy could be prepared with the help of laparoscopic surgery [10]; this makes the operation easier and spares the patient a painful perineotomy. Daniel Dargent designed the name of "coelio-Schauta" for this operation, which combines laparoscopy ("coelioscopie" according to the definition of the French pioneer Raoul Palmer) and a radical vaginal hysterectomy (Schauta operation). Different variants according to the blend of laparoscopic and vaginal surgery have recently been developed.

■ Routes for modified radical hysterectomy

Two major variants of modified radical hysterectomy using laparoscopic surgery have been described. The variant using laparoscopic surgery only will be referred to as the "full" laparoscopic MRH (LMRH) technique [10]. The variant combining a laparoscopic preparation with a radical vaginal hysterectomy will be referred to as the laparoscopic-vaginal MRH (LVRMH) technique, or "proximal coelio-Schauta".

In the first cases of laparoscopic modified radical hysterectomy (LMRH) presented in the literature, early (IA) cervical cancers were removed using a procedure reproducing abdominal modified radical hysterectomy. A pelvic lymphadenectomy was performed, with or without limited para-aortic node sampling. The ovarian, uterine and cervical pedicles were desiccated with bipolar current and divided with the carbon dioxide laser or with scissors. The ureters were unroofed, the rectovaginal and vesicovaginal spaces were developed, the parametria were divided laparoscopically. The vagina and some part of the remaining paracolpos were incised vaginally. Later on, a technique including laparoscopic incision of the vagina was described [10]. In these techniques, the laparoscopic approach effectively follows the steps of the technique used for laparotomy, the only basic difference being the way haemostasis is achieved. Bipolar cautery or stapling devices simply replace the clamps. The first videos presented by the pioneers of this technique were not really convincing, but later the team from Clermont Ferrand, France showed videos of indisputable radical hysterectomies.

LVMRH (proximal coelio-Schauta) is another concept. In the historical description of our operation (version 1), the uterine arteries were divided and the terminal ureters fully dissected laparoscopically; the operation was completed vaginally with the transection of the cardinal ligament and the placement of clamps on the cardinal ligament was made with the assumption that the ureters were displaced far enough from the operative field. However, our technique and a new version of our operation, differing on some points from the original technique, have evolved. At present, we feel the preparation of vaginal surgery by the opening of the lateropelvic spaces and the division of the uterine artery is sufficient in the majority of cases; as a consequence, we dissect the ureters vaginally, we pull the already divided uterine arteries out and we place the clamps on the cardinal ligaments under direct vision of the knee of the ureters. We give credit to Daniel Dargent for having taught us the technique of vaginal dissection of the ureter and to have imagined that uterine arteries could be simply pulled out vaginally after their laparoscopic division.

Whatever the blend of vaginal and laparoscopic techniques, the rationale of the coelio-Schauta procedure is that an oncological surgeon familiar with both laparoscopic surgery and radical vaginal hysterectomy is able to take advantage of the benefits of both routes in the same patient.

The advantages of laparoscopic surgery are:

– it is well suited to lymph node dissection;
– it gives direct access to the origin of the uterine arteries.

The drawbacks are:

– long operating time;
– blind vaginal incision.

Vaginal surgery:

– provides a precise incision of the vaginal cuff;
– ensures a modified radical hysterectomy with a minimum of operative time;
– has the unmatched advantage of a very limited dissection of the ureter.

Indeed, both routes may be used for the section of the parametria at the appropriate level, but the experienced vaginal surgeon will find the vaginal route shorter and requiring less ureteral dissection. In fact, the vaginal approach gives direct access to the middle part of the cardinal ligament, at the exact place where a clamp must be placed, and the ureter crosses the cardinal ligament exactly where the tip of the clamp must be placed. As a consequence, only a dissection of the ureter up to this point (the knee of the ureter being the most caudal point of the pelvic ureter) is required.

Combining the two approaches means combining advantages and eliminating drawbacks. In addition, starting surgery with the laparoscopic procedure makes vaginal surgery easier. The development of lateropelvic spaces improves uterine mobility, even if the cardinal ligaments are not divided laparoscopically. The laparoscopic division of the uterine artery ensures a relatively bloodless vaginal operative field. Both factors make identification of vaginal surgical planes and major landmarks easier, especially the knees of the ureters. The combination of the two minimal incision approaches may thus be the most logical technique for surgical therapy of cervical carcinomas in the future, avoiding the discomfort of both laparotomy and perineotomy, while reducing the excessively long operative time of laparoscopic surgery and adding accuracy to the placement of the vaginal incision.

Using concurrent laparoscopic and vaginal approaches requires choosing which step is best accomplished by each route. Lymphadenectomy can only be carried out by laparoscopy. The preferential use of either route for other steps may depend on the training of the surgeon or on individual features of the patient. The upper pedicles of the uterus (ovarian or utero-ovarian vessels) may be controlled laparoscopically or vaginally. Division of the uterine artery at its origin is more precisely accomplished laparoscopically. Laparoscopic unroofing of the ureter is unnecessary if no superficial uterine vein crosses the ureter with the uterine artery, as the latter will only have to be pulled vaginally. On the other hand, superficial uterine veins may bleed during the process of pulling the stump of the uterine artery from below and should be controlled laparoscopically, which means unroofing the ureter. Full dissection of the ureter in the vesicouterine ligament may be accomplished, as described below, laparoscopically or vaginally. Ureteral dissection is best performed vaginally by an experienced vaginal surgeon, but laparoscopic ureteral dissection may at times be easier than vaginal dissection in patients with a very narrow vagina. Finally, the very difference between LMRH and LVMRH is that the cardinal ligaments are divided laparoscopically in LMRH and vaginally in LVMRH.

■ Indications

The techniques of laparoscopic surgery may be applied to the treatment of cervical cancers at various stages

Simple hysterectomy or conisation alone is indicated in IA2 cervical cancers. For simple hysterectomy, the vaginal approach is the cheapest, shortest and safest route, compared to the abdominal or laparoscopic routes. When lymphadenectomy is indicated (depth of invasion between 3 and 5 millimetres or lymph vessel invasion), it may be performed laparoscopically in combination with vaginal hysterectomy or as a complement of a diagnostic conisation or simple hysterectomy.

Proximal (modified) radical hysterectomy is indicated for early invasive cervical cancer (IB tumour not exceeding 2 centimetres or 10 cm^3). This volume may be obtained after brachytherapy or the tumour may be small indicating a primary radical hysterectomy. Vaginal radical hysterectomy, laparoscopic radical hysterectomy or preferably the technique of laparoscopically-assisted radical vaginal hysterectomy (LARVH) with pelvic (interiliac) lymphadenectomy may be used. In our department, para-aortic dissection is only indicated in the pelvic positive-node patient.

Distal (classical) radical hysterectomy is indicated in larger but still non-bulky IB, IIA or proximal IIB tumours not previously submitted to radiation therapy. Vaginal procedures may be used for tumour volumes up to 4 centimetres or 50 cm^3. We advise the use of the distal (Dargent) type of LARVH or modified LARVH, combined with parametrial dissection if the pelvic and para-aortic lymphadenectomy does not yield positive nodes.

As bulky tumours (more than 4 centimetres or 50 cm^3) are not suitable for a primary vaginal approach, we use laparoscopic surgery only for staging in such cases.

When obviously diseased nodes are found, the question is whether to remove or to leave them for later irradiation. We feel that moderately enlarged nodes may be safely removed laparoscopically, provided they do not involve the iliac vessels. They must be dissected, not ruptured, and removed in an endoscopic bag. If a safe dissection cannot be performed laparoscopically, an extraperitoneal laparotomy is indicated.

References

[1] Childers J, Hatch K, Surwit E. The role of laparoscopic lymphadenectomy in the management of cervical carcinoma. *Gynecol Oncol* 1992 ; 47 : 38-43

[2] Dargent D. Laparoscopic surgery and gynecologic cancer. *Curr Opin Obstet Gynecol* 1993 ; 5 : 294-300

[3] Dargent D. Extraperitoneal aortic dissection. Award video presented at the Meeting of the Society of Gynecologic Oncologists, Phoenix, 1997

[4] Dargent D, Salvat J. L'envahissement ganglionnaire pelvien. Paris : Medsi/McGraw Hill, 1989

[5] Girardi F, Lichtenegger W, Tamussino K, Haas J. The importance of parametrial lymph nodes in the treatment of cervical cancer. *Gynecol Oncol* 1989 ; 34 : 206-211

[6] Haie C, Pejovic MH, Gerbaulet A, Horiot JC, Pourquier H, Delouche J et al. Is prophylactic para-aortic irradiation worthwhile in the treatment of advanced cervical carcinoma ? Results of a controlled clinical trial of the EORTC radiotherapy group. *Radiother Oncol* 1983 ; 11 : 101-112

[7] Kinney WK, Hodge DO, Egorshin EV, Ballard DJ, Podratz KC. Identification of a low-risk subset of patients with stage IB invasive squamous cancer of the cervix possibly suited to less radical surgical treatment. *Gynecol Oncol* 1995 ; 57 : 3-6

[8] Magrina JF, Goodrich MA, Weaver AL, Podratz KC. Modified radical hysterectomy: morbidity and mortality. *Gynecol Oncol* 1995 ; 59 : 277-282

[9] Michel G, Morice P, Castaigne D, Leblanc M, Rey A, Duvillard P. Lymphatic spread in stage Ib and II cervical carcinoma: anatomy and surgical implications. *Obstet Gynecol* 1998 ; 91 : 360-363

[10] Querleu D, Childers JM, Dargent D. Laparoscopic surgery in gynecologic oncology. Oxford : Blackwell Scientific, 1999

[11] Querleu D, Dargent D, Ansquer Y, Leblanc E, Narducci F. Extraperitoneal endosurgical aortic and common iliac dissection in the staging of bulky or advanced cervical carcinomas. *Cancer* 2000 ; 88 : 1883-1891

[12] Querleu D, Leblanc E. Laparoscopic infrarenal paraaortic lymph node dissection for restaging of carcinoma of the ovary or fallopian tube. *Cancer* 1994 ; 73 : 1467-1471

[13] Querleu D, Leblanc E, Castelain B. Laparoscopic pelvic lymphadenectomy in the staging of early cervical carcinoma. *Am J Obstet Gynecol* 1991 ; 164 : 579-581

[14] Rotman M, Pajak TF, Choi K, Clery M, Marcial V, Grigsby PW et al. Prophylactic extended-field irradiation of para-aortic lymph nodes in stages IIB and bulky IB and IIA cervical cancer. Ten-year treatment results of RTOG 79-20. *JAMA* 1995 ; 274 : 387-393

Chapter 11

Bulky stage I and II cervical carcinoma: a therapeutic dilemma

Tim Mould, John H Shepherd

T Mould, M.D.
Department of Gynaecological Oncology, University College London Hospital, London, United Kingdom.
JH Shepherd, M.D.
Department of Gynaecological Oncology, St Bartholomew's Hospital, East London Cancer Centre, Barts and The London NHS Trust, West Smithfield, London, United Kingdom.

Bulky stage I and II cervical carcinoma: a therapeutic dilemma

T Mould, JH Shepherd

Abstract. — *Lesion size is an independent predictor of survival in stage Ib and IIa carcinoma of the cervix with an increased risk of nodal metastases and local recurrence compared to tumours of smaller diameter. The treatment of bulky tumours is controversial. Traditionally, pelvic irradiation has been the treatment of choice, as both the central tumour and nodal metastases are treated using a single modality. Recent studies have reported improved results with concomitant chemoradiotherapy followed by extrafascial or radical hysterectomy for persistent disease. This should now be regarded as the treatment of choice. Surgery may be used as primary treatment in some clinical situations - young women with no evidence of metastatic or parametrial disease; the treatment of adenocarcinoma, where radiotherapy is less effective; the resection of bulky lymph node metastases. Surgery also provides accurate staging information so that the radiotherapy field may be extended to include the para-aortic area when the nodes are involved.*

Keywords: invasive carcinoma, bulky lymph nodes, radiotherapy, neoadjuvant chemotherapy, combined treatment.

Introduction

In women with stage Ib and IIa invasive carcinoma of the cervix, lesion size is an independent predictor of survival. Women with tumours of less than 2 cm in diameter have a 90% survival rate, whereas those with lesions greater than 2 cm have a 60% survival rate [32]. When the diameter of the tumour is greater than 4 cm the survival rate drops to 40% [7, 15].

Two factors account for the bad prognosis in larger cervical tumours. Firstly, local recurrence increases with lesion size. Patients with tumours greater than 6 cm in diameter have a 17.5% central failure rate when treated with radiotherapy alone [14]. Secondly, the incidence of lymph node metastases increases with the size of the tumour. Lymph node status is correlated closely with survival. Patients with negative nodes will have a 85-90% 5 year survival rate [10], whereas patients with positive nodes will have a survival rate varying between 20% and 74% depending on the number, size and site of the nodal metastases [3].

In view of these factors, the optimal treatment for large stage Ib and IIa cervical cancer is controversial. The commonly advocated treatment has been radiotherapy followed by extrafascial hysterectomy 6 weeks later. Recently reported studies indicate that concurrent chemoradiation is more effective than radiotherapy alone and that extrafascial hysterectomy may not be necessary, particularly for squamous cell carcinoma. The treatment for adenocarcinoma may prove to be different due to relative resistance to radiotherapy. There are centres using primary surgery to remove the central tumour, excise bulky nodal metastases and stage the disease, or laparoscopic surgery to stage the disease.

Radiotherapy

Pelvic irradiation had been the standard, definitive therapy for locally advanced cervical cancer as it treats both the central tumour and nodal metastases using a single treatment modality, thus keeping treatment morbidity to a minimum. External beam pelvic irradiation to a dose of 40-50 Gy over 4-5 weeks is followed by 2 intracavity implants boosting the dose to point A to a total of 80-90 Gy.

Two randomised studies of radiotherapy versus surgery for stage Ib carcinoma of the cervix have been reported. Newton reported a survival rate of 81% for radical surgery and 74% for radiotherapy [26]. The difference was not statistically significant.

Landoni et al randomised 343 women with stage Ib/IIa cervical cancer [21]. The groups were matched for nodal involvement as judged by lymphangiography. Overall survival and disease free survival was 83% and 74% respectively, and did not differ between the surgery and radiotherapy groups. The actuarial survival for the surgery and radiotherapy groups was 87% and 90% respectively for women with tumours less than 4 cm diameter, and 70% compared to 72% for women with tumours greater than 4 cm diameter. In the surgical group, 62 out of 114 women (54%) with tumours less than 4 cm, and 46 out of 55 women (84%) with tumours greater than 4 cm, received post-operative radiotherapy. Out of the 46 women who had adenocarcinoma, survival for the surgery group was superior to that of the radiotherapy group, 70% versus 59% ($P = 0.05$). Adenocarcinomas with a diameter greater than 4 cm were not analysed separately. Overall, for women with tumours greater than 4 cm, pelvic recurrence occurred in 16 out of 54 (29%) undergoing radiotherapy, and 9 out of 46 (19%) in the surgery group.

Thus radiotherapy is as effective as surgery for women with squamous cell carcinomas with a diameter greater than 4 cm. Furthermore, 84% of women in the surgical group also had adjuvant radiotherapy. Consequently the surgical group had a higher incidence of severe complications compared to the radiotherapy group, 28% versus 12% ($P = 0.0004$). Surgery was superior to radiotherapy in the treatment of adenocarcinoma (70% versus 59% survival respectively).

Concurrent chemoradiotherapy

Several phase II studies have reported that concomitant treatment with cisplatinum during radiotherapy results in faster and more complete responses plus better survival than expected with radiotherapy alone [6, 22, 23, 24]. Cisplatin potentiates the sublethal damage induced by radiotherapy and inhibits the repair of potentially lethal radiotherapy-induced damage [4, 35]. Keys et al reported a randomised controlled trial of radiotherapy versus radiotherapy plus concomitant cisplatin, with both arms followed by extrafascial hysterectomy, in 372 women with cervical tumours of 4 cm or more in diameter [20]. Women with evidence of involved lymph nodes were excluded. The pelvic irradiation field was set to extend 3 cm beyond the known extent of the disease and to encompass iliac and lower common iliac lymph nodes. The total irradiation dose was 45 Gy followed by one or two intracavity applications bringing the total dose to point A up to 75 Gy. In the chemotherapy group, cisplatin was given intravenously once a week at a dose of 40 mg/m² up to a maximum of 6 doses. Extrafascial hysterectomy was performed 3-6 weeks after completion of radiation.

Recurrence occurred in 37% of the radiation alone group and 21% of the combined cisplatinum/radiation group ($P < 0.001$), with a relative risk of recurrence of 0.51 (95% C.I. 0.43 - 0.75) in the combined group. Survival at 36 months median follow-up was significantly improved in the combined group with a relative risk of death of 0.54 (95% C.I. 0.34-0.86). The difference appeared to be due to a lower rate of relapse in the pelvic region. Thus concomitant chemotherapy improves the effectiveness of primary radiotherapy.

Combined treatment: radiotherapy/chemoradiotherapy plus surgery

In the study reported by Keys et al, there was residual cancer in the hysterectomy specimen in 48% of the combined group versus 59% of the radiotherapy alone group ($P = 0.04$) [20]. They quoted unpublished data showing that the overall risk of recurrence was not significantly reduced after hysterectomy - relative risk 0.76 (95% C.I. 0.52-1.12), despite a reduction in pelvic recurrence, and that survival was not significantly reduced - relative risk 0.91 after hysterectomy. Furthermore, hysterectomy adds considerable morbidity to the treatment [27]. They therefore suggested that hysterectomy following radiotherapy treatment was not necessary.

Traditional teaching has been that bulky tumours are especially prone to treatment failure with radiotherapy because of the large hypoxic tumour cell population. In addition, extension of the malignant growth into the adjacent portion of the myometrium and/or endometrium produces dosimetric problems, resulting in undertreatment of those areas. Rutledge et al reduced the incidence of central failure in cancers referred to as barrel-shaped endocervical lesions, by giving external radiation to shrink the tumour before administration of the intracavity therapy and by adding an adjuvant, extrafascial simple hysterectomy [30]. To minimise complications, they recommended no more than 40 Gy of whole pelvis radiation in four weeks and a single intracavity application. Survival at three years was improved in the hysterectomy group: 75% versus 64%. Gallion et al reduced the central recurrence rate in tumours with a diameter greater than 5 cm from 19% to 2% by addition of simple hysterectomy 4-6 weeks post radiation therapy [16]. Interestingly, extrapelvic recurrences were reduced in the hysterectomy group from 16% to 7%.

Due to the increased morbidity from surgery after radiotherapy and the conflicting evidence, a reasonable policy to adopt is to assess the cervix for persistent disease and a decision about hysterectomy is taken on the results. An examination under anaesthetic, punch biopsies, trucut biopsies and endocervical curettage should be performed three to six months after treatment. MRI is also useful to distinguish between radiotherapy changes and residual tumour. If small volume disease exists, an extrafascial hysterectomy may be performed, but if bulky disease is present a radical hysterectomy will be required.

Primary surgery

The high risk of requiring radiotherapy after primary surgery and thus subjecting the patient to the cumulative side effects of both treatment modalities means that primary surgery has not been the standard treatment for women with bulky cervical tumours. Primary surgery in bulky cervical tumour requires extensive dissection in order to ensure adequate clearance of the parametrium. The bladder, ureter and rectum need full mobilisation and thus the risk of surgical morbidity is high. As the chance of lymphovascular space involvement and perineural infiltration is increased with large tumours, adjunctive radiotherapy may be advisable in a significant proportion of cases despite adequate clearance. Adjunctive radiotherapy after radical surgery will further increase the risk of morbidity. Thus the reason for primary surgical treatment must be carefully considered before such therapy is undertaken.

However, there are situations where there is a role for primary surgery: young women; women with adenocarcinomas; women with bulky nodal metastases; and for surgically staging the disease either by laparotomy or using laparoscopic techniques.

■ Young women

Surgery has a role in young women with stage Ib and IIa disease where there is no evidence of parametrial or lymph node disease on examination under anaesthetic or MRI scan. In such cases, the risk of requiring adjunctive radiotherapy is approximately 20-25%. The preservation of ovarian and vaginal function and the reduction in long term morbidity that can be achieved with surgical treatment is important enough in this age group to warrant this level of risk.

■ Adenocarcinoma

The only randomised trial of surgery versus radiotherapy that included separate groups for squamous cell carcinoma and adenocarcinoma is the study by Landoni et al [21]. As described above, the survival for adenocarcinoma in the surgery and radiotherapy groups was 70% versus 59% respectively ($P = 0.05$). This study used radiotherapy alone and not combined chemoradiotherapy, but on the available evidence, surgery would be the favoured primary treatment in women with adenocarcinoma where there was no evidence of spread of disease outside the cervix.

■ Bulky lymph nodes

Surgery may be beneficial in women with bulky pelvic lymph node metastases. It has been estimated that 50 Gy will sterilise over 90% of microscopic nodal metastases, but not more than 50% of grossly involved lymph nodes [13]. To eradicate 90% of 2 cm nodes requires 60 Gy, and to eradicate 90% of nodes greater than 2 cm in diameter requires 70 Gy [36]. The pelvis is usually irradiated to 50 Gy, and generally not more than 60 Gy. Numerous studies have reported a poorer outcome in patients with macroscopically involved lymph nodes compared to patients with microscopically involved nodes [7, 19, 25]. However, three non-randomised studies have shown that women with resected bulky lymph nodes have the same survival curves as women with microscopically positive nodes [8, 11, 18]. Thus resection of bulky lymph nodes may have a therapeutic effect.

Adjunctive treatment had traditionally been postoperative radiotherapy for women with adverse prognostic factors such as lymph nodes metastases. A recent study has reported that concomitant chemoradiation is more effective than radiation alone in this situation [28]. This may alter the data above and mean that surgical debulking does not improve survival. A randomised trial would be needed to determine this.

■ Surgical staging

Clinical staging is accurate in approximately 60% of cases when compared to surgical staging, and undiagnosed lymph node involvement will be the cause of the error in many cases [1, 2]. The value of accurate staging depends on whether the treatment of metastatic disease beyond the standard radiation field will improve survival. A number of reports suggest some benefit from para-aortic radiotherapy. Patients who received radiation to the para-aortic region as part of initial treatment have been reported to have a survival advantage [5]. Patients found to have small volume para-aortic nodal disease at surgical staging and controllable pelvic disease may be cured with pelvic and para-aortic irradiation [9]. Treatment of unresected para-aortic nodes by extended field radiation led to long-term disease control in patients with low volume (less than 2 cm) nodal disease below L3 [34]. One study showed a survival advantage in patients with cervical tumours greater than 4 cm in diameter who received radiotherapy to the para-aortic nodes without any histological evidence of para-aortic disease [29]. A recent study using concomitant chemoradiation in women with para-aortic metastases reported overall survival of 50% for stage I, 39% stage II and 38% for stage III / IVa [33].

Toxicity of para-aortic radiotherapy is greater than pelvic radiation alone, but mostly was confined to patients with prior abdominal or pelvic surgery [29]. Retroperitoneal lymph node dissection produced fewer bowel complications than transperitoneal dissection [12, 29, 34]. In the combined chemoradiation study the late morbidity risk at 4 years was 14% and mostly involved the rectum [33].

Extended field treatment can therefore salvage patients with metastases outside the pelvis. Surgical dissection with histopathological analysis is the most accurate method of detecting para-aortic metastases.

■ Laparoscopic surgery

Surgical staging can be accomplished using laparoscopic techniques. Laparoscopic pelvic and para-aortic lymphadenectomy can be performed via a retroperitoneal approach. If the pelvic nodes are positive for metastatic tumour, radical radiotherapy is the treatment of choice. If the para-aortic nodes are positive, the radiotherapy field can be extended to include this area. This laparoscopic approach should reduce the morbidity of combined surgical and radiotherapy modalities, although there are no trials to confirm this. If the nodes are negative, there will be the option of performing radical surgery to clear the central tumour four to five days after lymphadenectomy.

Neoadjuvant chemotherapy

Chemotherapy has response rates of approximately 50% in squamous cell carcinoma of the cervix and has been evaluated as neoadjuvant therapy to shrink the tumour before surgery or radiotherapy in six randomised controlled trials [17]. Two trials showed significant benefit in survival, two showed no benefit and two showed a deleterious effect. One of the trials showing benefit reported the use of three courses of cisplatin-vincristine-bleomycin prior to surgery, plus adjuvant radiotherapy or primary radiotherapy in women with bulky stage I squamous cell carcinoma [31]. At median follow-up of 48 months, the chemotherapy arm had a superior progression free survival, 88% versus 67% ($P < 0.05$), and superior overall survival, 88% versus 70% ($P =$ not significant). It was reported that the operability had been improved and the parametrial extension had been decreased by neoadjuvant chemotherapy. They also reported a decrease in vascular embolism, lymph node involvement and tumour volume in the chemotherapy arm.

Thus neoadjuvant chemotherapy has a moderate response rate and significantly improved progression free survival. However, in view of the data on concurrent chemoradiation, the use of chemotherapy at the same time as radiation may be more beneficial.

References

[1] Averette HE, Dudan RC, Ford JH. Exploratory celiotomy for surgical staging of cervical cancer. *Am J Obstet Gynecol* 1972 ; 113 : 1090-1096

[2] Ballon SC, Berman ML, Lagasse LD, Petrilli ES, Castaldo TW. Survival after extraperitoneal pelvic and paraaortic lymphadenectomy and radiation therapy in cervical carcinoma. *Obstet Gynecol* 1981 ; 57 : 90-95

[3] Berek JS, Hacker NF. Practical gynecological oncology. Baltimore : Williams and Williams, 1994

[4] Carde P, Laval F. Effect of cis-dichlorodiammine platinum II and X rays on mammalian cell survival. *Int J Radiat Oncol Biol Phys* 1981 ; 7 : 929-933

[5] Carl UM, Bahnsen J, Wiegel T. Radiation therapy of para-aortic lymph nodes in cancer of the uterine cervix. *Acta Oncol* 1993 ; 32 : 63-67

[6] Chang HC, Lai CH, Chen MS, Chao AS, Chen LH, Soong YK. Preliminary results of concurrent radiotherapy and chemotherapy with cis-platinum, vincristine and bleomycin in bulky advanced cervical carcinoma: a pilot study. *Gynecol Oncol* 1992 ; 44 : 182-188

[7] Chung CK, Nahhas WA, Stryker JA, Curry SL, Abt AB, Mortel R. Analysis of factors contributing to treatment failures in stages IB and IIA carcinoma of the cervix. *Am J Obstet Gynecol* 1980 ; 138 : 550-556

[8] Cosin JA, Fowler JM, Chen MD, Paley PJ, Carson LF, Twiggs LB. Pretreatment surgical staging of patients with cervical carcinoma. *Cancer* 1998 ; 82 : 2241-2248

[9] Cunningham MJ, Dunton CJ, Corn B et al. Extended-field radiation therapy in early-stage cervical carcinoma: survival and complications. *Gynecol Oncol* 1991 ; 43 : 51-54

[10] Delgado G, Bundy B, Zaino R et al. Prospective surgical-pathological study of disease free interval in patients with stage Ib squamous cell carcinoma of the cervix: a Gynecological Oncology Group study. *Gynecol Oncol* 1990 ; 38 : 352-357

[11] Downey GO, Potish RA, Adcock LL, Prem KA, Twiggs LB. Pretreatment surgical staging in cervical carcinoma: therapeutic efficacy of pelvic lymph node resection. *Am J Obstet Gynecol* 1989 ; 160 : 1055-1061

[12] Fine BA, Hempling RE, Piver MS, Baker TR, McAuley M, Driscoll D. Severe radiation morbidity in carcinoma of the cervix: impact of pretherapy surgical staging and previous surgery. *Int J Radiat Oncol Biol Phys* 1995 ; 31 : 717-723

[13] Fletcher GH. Subclinical disease. *Cancer* 1984 ; 53 : 1274-1284

[14] Fletcher GH, Wharton JT. Principles of irradiation therapy for gynecologic malignancy. *Curr Probl Obstet Gynecol* 1978 ; 9 : 68

[15] Fuller AF Jr, Elliott N, Kosloff C, Hoskins WJ, Lewis JL Jr. Determinants of increased risk for recurrence in patients undergoing radical hysterectomy for stage Ib and IIa carcinoma of the cervix. *Gynecol Oncol* 1989 ; 33 : 34-39

[16] Gallion HH, Van Nagel JR Jr, Donaldson ES, Hanson M, Powell DE, Maruyama Y et al. Combined radiation therapy and extrafascial hysterectomy in the treatment of stage Ib barrel-shaped cervical cancer. *Cancer* 1985 ; 56 : 262-265

[17] Gibbs DD, Blake PR, Gore ME. Cytotoxic chemotherapy in the treatment of carcinoma of the uterine cervix. *Curr Obstet Gynaecol* 1999 ; 9 : 130-136

[18] Hacker NF, Wain GV, Nicklin JL. Resection of bulky positive lymph nodes in patients with cervical carcinoma. *Int J Gynecol Cancer* 1995 ; 5 : 250-256

[19] Husseinzadeh N, Shrake P, Deeulis T et al. Chemotherapy and extended field radiation therapy to para-aortic area in patients with histologically proven metastatic cervical cancer to para-aortic nodes: a phase II pilot study. *Gynecol Oncol* 1994 ; 52 : 326-331

[20] Keys HM, Bundy BN, Stehman FB, Muderspach LI, Chafe WE, Suggs CL et al. Cisplatin, radiation, and adjuvant hysterectomy compared with radiation and adjuvant hysterectomy for bulky stage Ib cervical carcinoma. *N Engl J Med* 1999 ; 340 : 1154-1161

[21] Landoni F, Maneo A, Colombo A et al. Randomised study of radical surgery versus radiotherapy for stage Ib-IIa cervical cancer. *Lancet* 1997 ; 350 : 535-540

[22] Lin J, Ho ES, Jan JS et al. High complete response rate of concomitant chemoradiotherapy for locally advanced squamous cell carcinoma of the uterine cervix. *Gynecol Oncol* 1996 ; 61 : 101-108

[23] Malfetano JH, Keys H, Kredentser D, Cunningham M, Kotlove D, Weiss L et al. Weekly cisplatin and radical radiation therapy for advanced, recurrent and poor prognosis cervical carcinoma. *Cancer* 1993 ; 71 : 3703-3706

[24] Malviya VK, Deppe G, Kim Y et al. Concurrent radiation therapy, cis-platinum, and mitomycin C in patients with poor prognosis cancer of the cervix: a pilot study. *Am J Clin Oncol* 1989 ; 12 : 434-437

[25] Monk BJ, Chan DS, Walker JL et al. Extent of disease as an indication for pelvic irradiation following radical hysterectomy and bilateral pelvic node dissection in the treatment of stage IB and IIA cervical carcinoma. *Gynecol Oncol* 1994 ; 54 : 4-9

[26] Newton M. Radical hysterectomy or radiotherpapy for stage I cervical cancer. *Am J Obstet Gynecol* 1975 ; 123 : 535-542

[27] O'Quinn AG, Fletcher GH, Wharton JT. Guidelines for conservative hysterectomy after irradiation. *Gynecol Oncol* 1980 ; 9 : 68-79

[28] Peters WA, Liu PY, Barret RJ et al. Cisplatin and 5-Fluorouracil plus radiation therapy are superior to radiation therapy as adjunctive in high-risk early stage carcinoma of the cervix after radical hysterectomy and pelvic lymphadenectomy: report of a phase III intergroup study. In *Society of Gynecologic Oncologist*, 1999

[29] Rotman M, Pajak TF, Choi K et al. Prophylactic extended-field irradiation of para-aortic lymph nodes in stages IIB and bulky IB and IIA: ten year treatment results of RTOG 79-20. *JAMA* 1995 ; 274 : 387-393

[30] Rutledge FN, Wharton JT, Fletcher GH. Clinical studies with adjunctive surgery and irradiation therapy in the treatment of carcinoma of the cervix. *Cancer* 1976 ; 38 : 596-602

[31] Sardi J, Sananes C, Giaroli A et al. Results of a prospective randomized trial with neoadjuvant chemotherapy in stage Ib, bulky squamous carcinoma of the cervix. *Gynecol Oncol* 1993 ; 49 : 156-165

[32] Van Nagel J, Donaldson E, Parker J et al. The prognostic significance of cell type and lesion size in patients with cervical cancer treated by radical surgery. *Gynecol Oncol* 1977 ; 5 : 142-151

[33] Varia MA, Bundy BN, Deppe G et al. Cervical carcinoma metastatic to para-aortic nodes: extended field radiation therapy with concomitant 5-fluorouracil and cisplatin chemotherapy: a gynecologic oncology group study. *Int J Radiat Oncol Biol Phys* 1998 ; 42 : 1015-1023

[34] Vigliotti AP, Wen BC, Hussey DH et al. Extended field irradiation for carcinoma of the uterine cervix with positive periaortic nodes. *Int J Radiat Oncol Biol Phys* 1992 ; 23 : 501-509

[35] Wallner KE, Li GC. Effect of cisplatin resistance on cellular radiation response. *Int J Radiat Oncol Biol Phys* 1987 ; 13 : 587-591

[36] Wharton JT, Jones HW 3rd, Day TG Jr, Rutledge FN, Fletcher GH. Preirradiation celiotomy and extended field irradiation for invasive carcinoma of the cervix. *Obstet Gynecol* 1977 ; 49 : 333-338

Chapter 12

Treatment of cervical carcinoma stages III and IV

Pierluigi Benedetti Panici, Giuseppe Cutillo, Francesco Maneschi,
Mariangela Amoroso, Mario Congiu, Innocenza Palaia

P Benedetti Panici, M.D.
G Cutillo, M.D.
F Maneschi, M.D.
M Amoroso, M.D.
M Congiu, M.D.
I Palaia, M.D.
Department of Gynaecology, Campus Biomedico, Libera Universita, via E. Longoni 83, Rome, Italy.

Treatment of cervical carcinoma stages III and IV

P Benedetti Panici, G Cutillo, F Maneschi, M Amoroso, M Congiu, I Palaia

Abstract. — *Clinical management of locally-advanced cervical carcinoma represents a therapeutic challenge for gynaecological oncologists, radiotherapists and medical oncologists. Despite screening programmes and reliable methods for early detection, in about one-fourth of all cases, carcinoma of the cervix is still diagnosed at stages III and IV. Radiotherapy is the current standard of treatment for women at stage III-IVA, while palliative therapies only are indicated for stage IVB patients. Over recent decades, thanks to advances in radiotherapeutic techniques, significant improvements in 5-year survival rates have been observed in stage III patients. However, the long-term outcome and morbidity of radiotherapy is still a major issue, and the 5-year probability that these women will be alive and free of moderate and severe morbidity is disappointing. In recent years, new, integrated therapeutic strategies have been tested in the treatment of locally-advanced cervical carcinoma. The results of different randomised trials seem to indicate that concurrent chemotherapy and radiotherapy and neoadjuvant chemotherapy, followed by radical surgery, are the most promising in this clinical setting. However, longer follow-up and confirmatory studies are needed before introducing these novel therapeutic approaches into clinical practice. Platinum-based chemotherapy and radiotherapy are both effective for symptomatic palliation of stage IVB patients. Clinical complaints as well as quality-of-life issues should be taken into account when deciding upon the therapeutic approach in this incurable group of patients.*

Keywords: advanced cervical cancer, integrated therapies, radiotherapy.

Introduction

According to the FIGO (International Federation of Gynaecology and Obstetrics) staging system, cervical carcinoma at stages III and IV comprises a heterogeneous group of locally-advanced tumours, including both gross loco-regional spread of disease (involving the vagina, parametria, bladder and/or rectum) and overt, distant metastases (peritoneum, lung, liver, bones, etc.). Consequently, the clinical management as well as the prognosis of these women are completely different, there being patients still amenable to definitive treatment and cure (stages III and IVA) and others who can only benefit from palliative therapies (stage IVB). For clarity, this distinction will be pursued in this chapter, which will review the current modalities of treatment of cervical carcinoma at stages III and IV.

Epidemiology and Staging

Carcinoma of the cervix is the third most common tumour in women worldwide, after breast and colon cancer [29]. Despite screening programmes and reliable methods for early detection, cervical cancer is diagnosed at stage III and IV in 21% and 4% of patients, respectively [1]. These percentages are likely to be even higher in developing countries, where cervical carcinoma is the leading cause of death among women (80% of cancer cases diagnosed yearly), and where a worse overall survival is observed (average 5-year survival rate: Developing Countries 49%, Europe 59%, USA 69%) [29].

Carcinoma of the cervix is the only gynaecological tumour clinically staged. According to FIGO rules, pre-treatment work-up should consist of: pelvic examination under anaesthesia, cystoscopy, proctoscopy, excretory urography, skeletal radiography, barium enema and chest X-rays. As shown *(table I)*, the probability of positive results at imaging assessment increases with the clinical stage [38]. However, in the absence of specific symptoms (tenesmus, dysuria, difficult voiding, etc.), signs (rectorrhagia, haematuria, etc.) and findings at physical examination (involvement of the vesico-vaginal or recto-vaginal septum, gross parametrial involvement), the diagnostic yield from routine evaluation of the gastrointestinal and urological tract is very low. There is good evidence that an individualisation of staging procedures based on clinical presentation of the disease can be equally effective in assessing loco-regional tumour spread, determining a significative saving of time, cost and potential morbidity [19].

Table I. Positive findings at imaging evaluation according to FIGO stage (modified by Russel [38]).

Type of examination	IB-IIA	IIB-IVA	IVB
Chest radiography	0.7 %	2.1 %	30.1 %
Pyelography	4.4 %	22.2 %	47.5 %
Barium enema	2.8 %	9.1 %	24.6 %
Bone scan	2.2 %	4.7 %	46.3 %
CT	43.2 %	74.5 %	88.5 %
MRI	52.1 %	76.6 %	87.5 %
Lymphangiography	21.2 %	52.0 %	93.8%

Table II. Laparoscopic abdominal staging: histologically confirmed peritoneal spread according to FIGO stage and histotype [3].

FIGO STAGE	Squamous carcinoma	Squamous positive patients	Adeno-carcinoma	Adeno-positive patients	Total cases	Total positive patients
IB-IIA > 4 cm	8	2 (25 %)	1	-	9	2 (33%)
IIB	20	2 (10 %)	1	-	21	2 (10 %)
III	13	5 (38 %)	3	1	16	6 (37 %)
IVA	9	5 (55 %)	1	-	10	5 (50 %)
Total	50	14 (28 %)	6	1	56	15 (27 %)

Knowledge of the nodal status and of the site of lymphatic metastasis are both very important for planning the primary treatment of advanced cervical tumours. Dose and field of irradiation, as well as the need for debulking nodal surgery, are decided mainly on these clinical findings. Therefore, radiological evaluation of retroperitoneal disease is routinely performed in the management of locally-advanced cervical carcinoma. However, given the suboptimal sensitivity of both CT scan and MRI in detecting microscopic nodal disease, surgical evaluation of aortic nodes is performed in many centres in order to select patients for either extended field irradiation or systemic therapy. Pathologically-negative aortic nodes are required for entry into several research protocols of the G.O.G. (Gynaecologic Oncology Group) on locally-advanced cervical carcinoma.

Abdominal spread of cervical cancer is present in about 10-50% of patients with locally-advanced disease *(table II)* [5]. Whatever the therapy, the prognosis of these patients is very poor, less than 20% of them being long-term survivors [16]. Therefore, pre-treatment evaluation of abdominal status could be useful for selecting patients not amenable to curative treatment, avoiding the morbidity of either full-dose radiotherapy or radical surgery. Laparoscopy has proven to be a reliable and minimally-invasive technique in assessing the intraperitoneal spread of locally-advanced cervical cancer [5]. However, further studies are needed to evaluate the potential benefits of intra-abdominal laparoscopic staging in this clinical setting.

Therapy of stages III-IVA

■ Radiotherapy

Primary radiotherapy consisting of external pelvic irradiation, followed by intracavitary brachytherapy, is the current standard of treatment of cervical carcinoma at FIGO stages III-IVA. According to the last Annual Report, the 5-year survival rate of locally-advanced patients treated exclusively by radiotherapy was 36.3% at stage IIIA, 41.7% at stage IIIB and 16.4% at stage IVA [1]. Over the years, thanks to advances in radiotherapeutic techniques, remarkable improvements in 5-year survival rates have been observed in stage III patients (1973: 25%, 1978: 39%, 1983: 47%) [22]. However, the long-term morbidity of radiotherapy is still a major issue. Indeed, the probability that locally-advanced patients will survive without tumour recurrence and moderate or severe morbidity is disappointing *(table III)* [30].

In a retrospective analysis performed at M.D. Anderson on more than 1,000 patients with stage IIIB cervical tumours, Longsdon and Eifel have identified by multivariate

Table III. Five-year actuarial probabilities of being alive, cured and free from late combined organ* morbidity in relation to FIGO stage (modified by Pedersen [30]).

FIGO STAGE	Moderate morbidity	Severe morbidity
IIB	22 ± 4	36 ± 4
IIIB	9 ± 2	17 ± 3
IVA	3 ± 2	7 ± 3

*: Rectosigmoideum, bladder, small intestine, ureters and vagina/portio/uterus.

Table IV. Incidence and prognostic significance of clinical characteristics in 983 stage III patients treated with curative intent (modified by Longsdon and Eifel [24]).

Characteristics	No. patients (%)	DSS (%)	p
Age			0.0003
< 40	133 (14)	29	
≥ 40	850 (86)	38	
Weight loss			0.03
< 10 %	854 (87)	37	
≥ 10 %	129 (13)	34	
Pain at diagnosis			0.96
present	302 (31)	39	
absent	681 (69)	36	
Pretreatment haemoglobin level			0.0002
≥ 10 g/dL	702 (74)	39	
< 10 g/dL	249 (26)	30	
Lowest haemoglobin level during RT			< 0.0001
≥ 10 g/dL	505 (53)	44	
< 10 g/dL	441 (47)	29	

DSS: disease-specific survival rate at 5 years.

analysis clinical characteristics and tumour-related factors affecting disease-specific survival of women treated with radiotherapy with curative intent *(tables IV, V)* [24]. Besides these unmodifiable clinical prognosticators, however, some technical aspects of radiotherapeutic treatment have been shown to be of utmost importance for successful treatment of locally-advanced cervical carcinoma:

– duration of treatment;

– performance of brachytherapy;

– total central dose (dose at point A);

– radiation field design and extent.

Table V. Incidence and prognostic significance of tumour-related factors in 983 stage III patients treated with curative intent (modified by Longsdon and Eifel [24]).

Characteristics	No. patients (%)	* DSS (%)	p
Extent of tumor			< 0.0001
No pelvic wall involvement	54 (5)	34	
Fixed to one pelvic wall	414 (42)	44	
One pelvic wall + opposite lateral parametrium	253 (26)	35	
Fixed to both pelvic walls	262 (27)	27	
Clinical tumour diameter			0.0001
< 6 cm	35	59	
6-7.9 cm	97	48	
> 8 cm	282	30	
Hydronephrosis			< 0.0001
absent	682 (70)	40	
present	291 (30)	28	
Lower third vagina			0.0001
not involved	866 (88)	38	
involved	117 (12)	25	
Lymphangiogram**			0.001
Entirely negative	288 (53)	43	
External iliac nodes	119 (22)	30	
Common iliac nodes	54 (10)	25	
Paraortic nodes	30 (5)	23	
Equivocal findings	56 (10)	28	
Pelvic wall fixation after 40-45 Gy**			< 0.0001
No	188 (19)	52	
Yes	657 (67)	33	

* DSS: disease-specific survival rate at 5 years
** Lymphangiogram was obtained in 547/983 patients (53%). Categories represent the highest level of involvement
*** The reponse of pelvic wall disease was not described in 138 cases.

Since these factors are mainly operator-dependent, their clinical importance will be briefly addressed.

In the literature, there is mounting evidence that protraction of treatment may significantly worsen the clinical outcome of patients with locally-advanced cervical carcinoma [12, 13, 23, 34]. A highly significant increase in pelvic relapse was observed by Lanciano when total treatment time was increased from less than 6 weeks to more than 10 weeks (actuarial 4-year pelvic recurrence rate: 5% vs 20%, $P = 0.0001$) [23]. This trend was particularly evident for stage III patients in terms of both local control rate (4.3% vs 42.4%) and absolute survival (70.6% vs 30.4%), respectively. At multivariate analysis, total treatment time continued to be an independent prognosticator for infield recurrence (P = 0.003), together with stage (P < 0.0001) and age (P = 0.01). Similar results were reported by Petereit in 209 patients with cervical carcinoma at stage IB-IIIB [34]. In this study, the median treatment duration was 55 days: when all patients were subdivided into those treated in less than 55 days and those who took 55 or more days to complete treatment, survival was significantly better in the shorter treatment time group (5-years survival 65% vs 54%, P = 0.03). In particular, in stage III patients a shorter treatment duration (< 55 days) determined both a better survival (52% vs 42%) and pelvic control rate (76% vs 55%). Major late complications were not influenced by treatment time. A linear decrease of loco-regional control and survival, amounting to approximately 1% per day of prolonged treatment, has been observed by Fyles and Girinsky [12, 13]. These data should be interpreted cautiously, because patients with more advanced tumours and concomitant clinical problems are more often treated over a longer overall time, and studies comparing continuous and split-course radiotherapy have clearly shown that treatment prolongation should be avoided [31]. Therefore, the current recommendation is to try complete external and intracavitary treatment in as short a time as possible, avoiding treatment interruption. Patients should be given dietary instructions and medication to avoid intestinal toxicity accompanied by diarrhoea, which is the most common cause of interruption of treatment [19].

The use of brachytherapy is the most important predictor of treatment success, even more than external dose, intracavitary dose, or the number of implant applications a patient receives [19]. In a retrospective analysis at M.D. Anderson, the 5-year disease-specific survival of patients at stage IIIB who completed treatment with curative intent was 45% when intra-cavitary therapy (ICRT) was performed and 24% when ICRT was not performed (P < 0.0001) [24]. An indirect confirmation of the importance of brachytherapy in locally-advanced cervical tumours was reported by Komaki et al [22]. These authors, analysing the results of the Patterns of Care Study, reported a significant improvement in the local/pelvic control rate in stage III patients treated in 1983, when compared with those treated in earlier periods (1973: 37%, 1978: 49%, 1983: 69%, P = 0.03). During the same years, a parallel increase in the percentage of patients receiving both brachytherapy (1973: 60%, 1983: 88%) and a higher energy of external pelvic irradiation (1973: 28%, 1983: 87%) was observed. As the mean lateral pelvic dose remained constant over the three periods, the authors concluded that the increase in mean paracentral dose and tumour pelvic control observed in stage III patients was mainly due to a more frequent use of brachytherapy in recent years rather than to higher energy linear accelerators. Despite this evidence, the results of a recent survey of the American Brachytherapy Society have shown that only 60% of radiotherapists utilise brachytherapy for the treatment of carcinoma of the cervix [26]. These percentages are likely to be even lower in locally-advanced patients, where both distortion of the anatomy due to tumour spread and narrowing of the vagina by external radiotherapy can prevent the routine insertion of regular applicators and ovoids.

Total dose to point A seems to be crucial for local control of disease: in stage IIIB-IVA patients, a central dose of 85-90 Gy should be delivered [19]. About 40-50 Gy are given by external pelvic irradiation, while the remainder are delivered with intracavitary implants. A correlation between paracentral doses and central disease control was described by Perez et al in a group of 128 women with bulky tumour of the cervix: no pelvic relapses were observed in the group of patients receiving more than 80 Gy, while pelvic failure rates of 13% and 15% were reported in the groups receiving 60-80 Gy and < 60 Gy, respectively [33]. A similar experience has been reported at M.D. Anderson in

98 patients with cervical carcinoma of more than 6 cm in diameter: the 5-year pelvic recurrence rate was 33% for women receiving less than 85-90 Gy to point A, and 16% for those receiving higher paracentral doses ($P = 0.03$) [11].

The importance of using the appropriate external beam irradiation field in the treatment of locally-advanced cervical carcinoma has been recently pointed out by Greer [15]. Traditionally, pelvic radiation portals have been based on radiographically-visualised skeletal landmarks. However, recent studies based on intraoperative measurements [14], magnetic resonance imaging [39], computed tomography [21] and lymphangiography [32] have shown the potential pitfalls of using traditional external-beam irradiation fields in the treatment of cervical cancer, with the potential to miss the gross tumour or pathways of parametrial (i.e. posterior attachment of the utero-sacral and cardinal ligaments) and nodal spread (i.e. common iliac and upper external iliac nodes). As this can lead to an increase in local failure [21], careful attention to pelvic external-beam irradiation design is needed to complement brachytherapy in locally-advanced patients.

Aortic nodal metastases are present in about 30-40% of patients with locally-advanced cervical carcinoma [48]. Most of these metastases are microscopic or undetected by standard radiological diagnostic techniques. Thus, the aortic area, unless macroscopically involved, is not included in the radiation treatment fields. However, a randomised trial of RTOG, comparing pelvic radiotherapy with prophylactic extended-field irradiation of para-aortic lymph nodes in high risk patients with cervical carcinoma, has shown a significant survival advantage in the extended-field irradiation arm (10 year overall survival: 55% vs 44%, $P = 0.02$) [37]. When macroscopic nodal metastases are found (bulky nodes), the ability of radiotherapy to sterilise nodal disease, without serious morbidity, is very low. In this setting, surgical debulking of nodal disease by an extraperitoneal route prior to radiation therapy has been shown to be effective. A similar survival for patients with completely resected lymph nodes was observed, whether they were microscopically or macroscopically positive [9]. Remarkably, no increase in treatment-related morbidity or mortality was reported through the combination of extraperitoneal surgical staging and radiotherapy.

■ Concurrent chemotherapy and radiotherapy

The concomitant administration of chemotherapy with radiotherapy has proved helpful in a variety of tumour sites, including the head and neck, bladder and anus. Since 1985, the Gynecologic Oncologic Group has considered chemo-radiation with hydroxyurea the standard treatment for patients with locally-advanced cervical carcinoma [18]. However, this treatment modality has never gained wide diffusion in the gynaecological community. A renewed interest in concurrent chemotherapy and radiotherapy has recently emerged following the results of four large-scale randomised clinical trials which have shown the superiority of cisplatin-based chemo-radiation over both radiotherapy alone and radiotherapy plus hydroxyurea in the treatment of locally-advanced cervical carcinoma [20, 25, 36, 49] *(table VI)*. Even though a stage-for-stage survival analysis was not reported in these papers, a survival benefit for stage III-IVA patients may be supposed (this represents one-third to half of the patients entered into these trials). Not surprisingly, these improvements in outcome were won at the expense of increased short-term toxicity, whereas no obvious increase in long-term side effects was observed. The promising results of these studies prompted the National Cancer Institute to issue a clinical announcement suggesting that "strong consideration should be given to the incorporation of concurrent cisplatin-based chemotherapy with radiation therapy in women who require radiation therapy for treatment of cervical cancer." In

Table VI. Concurrent chemotherapy and radiotherapy: literature review.

Study	Stage	Standard treatment	Experimental treatment	Overall survival	RR
Keys [20]	IB2	Radiotherapy	RT + weekly CDDP	72 % vs 86 %	0.54
Morris [25]	IB2-IVA	Extended-field radiotherapy	RT + CDDP, 5-FU	58 % vs 73 %	0.52
Rose [36]	IIB-IVA	Radiotherapy + HU	RT + weekly CDDP and	36 % vs 68 %	0.61
			RT + CDDP + 5-FU + HU	36 % vs 66 %	0.58
Whitney [49]	IIB-IVA	Radiotherapy + HU	RT + CDDP, 5-FU	52 % vs 62 %	0.74

RT: radiotherapy; HU: hydroxyurea; CDDP: cisplatin. RR: relative risk.

consideration of the limited follow-up period and of the sub-optimal results obtained in the control arm group in some of these studies [25, 36] (which could partially explain the significant improvement of survival observed in the concurrent chemo-radiation group), we believe that more mature data are needed before considering this novel therapeutic approach as the new standard in the treatment of locally-advanced cervical carcinoma.

■ Sequential chemotherapy and radiotherapy

Unlike concurrent chemotherapy and radiation, where radio-sensitising properties of cytotoxic agents are utilised, administration of chemotherapy in the neoadjuvant setting has two main objectives: treating distant micrometastasis and reducing tumour bulk before definitive treatment. In the last decade, a number of randomised studies comparing radiotherapy with sequential chemotherapy and radiotherapy in locally-advanced cervical tumours were carried out *(table VII)*. None of these trials has reported improved results in terms of tumour control rate, time-to-disease progression, or survival in the experimental group. An even worse outcome in patients treated with combined therapy was observed in the studies of Tattersall and Souhami, this group having also been prematurely closed due to an unacceptable toxicity in the chemotherapy arm (four treatment-related deaths) [43, 47]. Various hypotheses have been proposed to explain the unsatisfactory results observed: accelerated repopulation of tumour clonogens caused by neoadjuvant chemotherapy; delay in initiation of radiotherapy by neoadjuvant chemotherapy; low statistical power of published studies; tumour heterogeneity, etc. [35]. Currently, due to the lack of demonstrated clinical benefit, sequential chemotherapy and radiotherapy should be discouraged in the treatment of locally-advanced cervical carcinoma.

■ Neoadjuvant chemotherapy followed by radical surgery

Historically, surgery has had little or no role in the primary treatment of locally-advanced cervical carcinoma, and apart from a period of renewed popularity during the 1950s, it has usually been reserved for the treatment of early disease. Unacceptable perioperative mortality, high prevalence of major morbidity, and technical difficulties with respect to the basic principle of oncological surgery (namely, not cutting through the tumour) have caused it to fall into disuse in patients with advanced stage disease. Recently, the surgical treatment of locally-advanced cervical carcinoma has been regaining acceptance [2, 10, 42]. There are several reasons to explain this new trend. Improvements in anaesthesia and perioperative care have been dramatic, reducing perioperative mortality to less than 1% [17]. The introduction of neoadjuvant

Table VII. Randomised trials of neoadjuvant chemotherapy (NACT) followed by radiotherapy (RT) versus RT alone: literature review.

Author	Stage	Pts	Regimen (cycles)	Clinical Resp.(%)		Survival		p
				NACT + RT	RT	NACT + RT	RT	
Cardenas (1993)	IIIB	28	PEC (4)	45	86	36 % **	50 % **	-
Chauvergne (1993)	IIB-III	151	MCVP (2-4)	96	93	40 % **	35 % **	NS
Kumar (1994)	IIB-IVA	177	BIP (2)	70	69	38 % * 70 % **	43 %* 68 % **	NS
Souhami (1992)	IIIB	91	VBMP (3)	47	32	23 % *	39 % *	0.02
Sundfor (1996)	IIIB-IVA	94	P5FU (3)	56	61	32 %*	37 %*	NS
Tattersal (1995)	IIB-IVA	260	PE (3)	43	65	49 %*	70 %*	0.02
Tobias (1990)	IIA-IVA	66	BIP (3)	75	56	-	-	-

* Overall survival; ** DFS.

Table VIII. Phase II studies of neoadjuvant chemotherapy followed by surgery: literature review.

Author	Pts	Stage	Regimen (cycles)	% CR (cCr)	% Op	% pCR
Benedetti Panici (1998)	128	IB2-III	PB ± M (1-3)	83 (15)	76	18
Bloss (1995)	30	IIB-IVA	PVB (3)	87 (0)	34	0
Carlos do Valle (1992)	21	III-IVA	CPA (3-5)	67 (14)	67	-
Deppe (1991)	17	IB-IIIB	PmitC (3)	76 (29)	59	20
Dottino (1991)	28	IB-IVA	PVBM (1)	100 (35)	93	15
Kirsten (1987)	47	IB-IVA	PVB (3)	66 (11)	32	0
Lacava (1997)	42	IIB-IVA	VNB (12 weeks)	45 (5)	32	0
Leone (1996)	57	IIB-IVA	PI (3)	54 (7)	48	7
Sardi (1990)	151	IIB-III	PVB (3)	86 (22)	62	na
Zanetta (1998)	38	IB2-IVA	TIP (3)	84 (29)	89	16

CR: clinical response; cCR: complete clinical response; Op: operability; pCR: pathological complete response.

chemotherapy, by inducing regression of cervical tumour and its local spread, has made radical surgery feasible in most locally-advanced patients [2]. Surgical improvements, such as the vessel-by-vessel resection of the lateral parametrium with hemoclips, as well as new techniques for the dissection of the cervicovesical ligament and prevention of ureteral fistulas, have made it possible to entirely remove the pericervical tissue with acceptable morbidity [4, 8]. Thorough removal of the pelvic and aortic nodes draining the cervix has been proven to be feasible [6].

Thanks to these advances, in the last decade various pilot studies investigating the feasibility and efficacy of neoadjuvant chemotherapy followed by radical surgery in locally-advanced cervical cancer were carried out *(table VIII)*. Substantially, these studies have shown that preoperative chemotherapy makes radical surgery possible in most advanced patients without increasing perioperative morbidity [4] *(table IX)*. Moreover,

Table IX. Operative morbidity following neoadjuvant chemotherapy and type IV-V radical hysterectomy in stage III patients [4].

No. Patients	42
Intraoperative complications	
Severe haemorrhage (> 1 500 mL)	2 (5 %)
Ureteral injury	1 (3 %)
Bladder injury	1 (3 %)
Rectal injury	1 (3 %)
Postoperative complications	
Lymphocyst	14 (33 %)
Pulmonary embolism	3 (7 %)
Deep venous thrombosis	4 (9 %)
Ureteral fistula	3 (7 %)
Laparocele	3 (7 %)

Table X. Randomised trials of neoadjuvant chemotherapy followed by radical surgery.

Author	Stage	Pts	Arm	Overall Survival	p
Sardi (1996)	IIIB	150	NACT + RS + RT	63 %	0.005 [1]
			NACT + RT	53 %	0.02 [2]
			RT	37 %	
Sardi (1998)	IIB	295	NACT + RS	65 %	0.005 [3]
			NACT + RT	54 %	0.001 [4]
			RT	48 %	
			RS	41 %	
Benedetti Panici (1999)	IB2-III	441	NACT + RS	59 %	0.007
			RT	44 %	

NACT: neoadjuvant chemotherapy; RT: radiotherapy; RS: radical surgery.
(1): NACT + RS + RT versus RT.
(2): NACT + RT versus RT.
(3): NACT + RS versus RT.
(4): NACT + RS versus RS.

an improvement in survival (when compared with the results of the historical series) was observed in some of these studies [2, 10, 42]. It should be noted that the clinical response to neoadjuvant chemotherapy turned out to be one of the most important predictors of survival at multivariate analysis [7]. However, a complete pathological response was observed only in a small percentage of these patients, residual disease having been found both alone and concomitantly at the level of the cervix, vagina, parametria and lymph nodes [4]. Hence, the authors concluded that due to the unpredictable pattern of tumour response to chemotherapy, every surgical effort should be made in these operable patients to avoid leaving residual disease and to achieve the best chances of cure.

On the basis of the encouraging results obtained in phase II studies, different randomised trials comparing neoadjuvant chemotherapy, followed by surgery with standard radiotherapy, have been carried out in recent years [3, 40, 41] *(table X)*. In all these studies, experimental therapy has been shown to be superior to standard radiotherapy. Stage III patients were included in only two of these trials, which will be briefly discussed. In 1996, Sardi et al [40] reported the results of a prospective randomised study in stage III patients with cervical carcinoma comparing three different therapies:

– radiotherapy only (54 patients);

– neoadjuvant chemotherapy followed by radiotherapy (54 patients);

– neoadjuvant chemotherapy followed by surgery and whole pelvic irradiation (53 patients).

Clinical response to neoadjuvant chemotherapy was similar in both the experimental arms; and the operability rate in the chemo-surgical group was 73%. A significant improvement of survival was observed in both groups receiving neoadjuvant chemotherapy when compared with standard radiotherapy *(table X)*. Patients with hydronephrosis or bilateral parametrial involvement had the worst outcome. In this subset of patients, no significant differences were found among the three treatment arms, even though neoadjuvant chemotherapy followed by surgery produced the best survival rates. Neoadjuvant chemotherapy determined a better local control of disease (pelvic recurrence rate: exclusive RT 50%, neoadjuvant CT followed by RT 32%, neoadjuvant CT followed by surgery 18%, $P < 0.001$), while no significant differences were observed in distant recurrence rates.

In 1990, an Italian multicentric randomised trial was undertaken to compare the efficacy and toxicity of sequential neoadjuvant chemotherapy and radical surgery, versus only radiation therapy in locally-advanced cervical cancer (FIGO stage IB2-III) [3]. Of the 441 patients selected, 409 received the treatment as assigned. Radical surgery was feasible in 55% of stage III patients, compared with 85.5% of those presenting with less advanced disease ($P < 0.0001$). Both treatments were well tolerated and, despite an increased but reversible haematological toxicity due to chemotherapy, long-term complication rates were similar in the two groups. A significant improvement of both overall and progression-free survival was reported in the experimental arm *(table X)*. This result was further confirmed at multivariate analysis where type of treatment as well as FIGO stage, pre-operative nodal status, tumour size and institution were all independent prognostic factors [3]. Survival analysis by FIGO stage revealed a significant improvement for stage IB2-IIB patients (5-year overall survival: 65% versus 46%, $p = 0.05$; 5-year progression-free survival: 60% versus 47%, $P = 0.02$), but only a trend was observed for stage III (5-year overall survival: 41% versus 37%, $P = 0.36$; 5-year progression-free survival: 42% versus 36%, $P = 0.29$). In this study, unlike the Argentine trial, postoperative radiotherapy was not routinely administered.

In conclusion, radical surgery appears to be a feasible option in chemosensitive women with locally-advanced cervical cancer. Survival results seem to be comparable, if not superior, to radiotherapy, while long-term morbidity appears favourable. Given these results, coupled with those recently obtained using concurrent chemotherapy and radiotherapy in United States [20, 25, 36, 49], we believe that a randomised study comparing neoadjuvant chemotherapy followed by surgery with concurrent chemo-radiation is warranted.

Table XI. Symptomatic palliation with large single-dose-monthly interval schedule (literature review).

Author	No of patients	Bleeding	Pain
Halle (1986)	32	44 %	50 %
Hodson (1983)	14	64 %	21 %
Spanos (1987)	5	58 %	

Table XII. Symptomatic palliation with accelerated split-course schedule [45].

Symptom	No of patients presenting with symptom	% totally cleared
Dysuria	9	67
Pain	36	31
Ulceration	14	50
Bleeding	49	76
Constipation	7	43
Tenesmus	4	100

Therapy of stage IVB

Cervical carcinoma at stage IVB is an incurable disease, the median survival and 5-year survival rate of these patients being 8 months and 10%, respectively [1]. Thus, palliation of symptoms and prolongation of survival should be the main objectives of therapy. Palliation can be loco-regional or systemic in nature and can be performed by chemotherapy, radiotherapy and surgery (in a few selected cases). The choice of treatment must take into account the pattern of spread of the disease and the clinical complaints of the patient. Cervical carcinoma has a propensity to progress loco-regionally and to produce symptoms by distant metastasis (dyspnea, bone pain, subocclusive symptoms, etc.) only late in the natural history of tthe disease. Therefore, palliation of pelvic disease is the main challenge for clinicians.

Radiotherapy has proven to be effective in symptomatic palliation of pelvic disease [45]. Two different palliation schemes can be utilised:

– the large single dose (10 Gy delivered at monthly intervals to a maximum dose of 30 Gy) [46];

– the accelerated split course (3.7 Gy per fraction given twice a day to a total dose of 44.4 Gy) [44].

Both schedules offer substantial symptomatic palliation *(tables XI, XII)*, are compact, cause minimal acute toxicity (3-4% of G1-G2 toxicity on the bladder and rectum) and require little commitment of patient time. However, a remarkable higher long-term toxicity is observed with the large single dose scheme (12-month actuarial toxicity: 42% vs 7%). Hence, when patient life expectancy is more than 6 months, the accelerated split-course schedule should be preferred.

In the literature, no systematic study of chemotherapy on naive patients with stage IVB has been performed. Thus, only indirect evidence is available on the efficacy of chemotherapy palliation in this clinical setting. These derive both from studies of neoadjuvant chemotherapy in earlier stages of the disease, and from the experience with extra-pelvic recurrences in pretreated patients. It is well established that in naive patients with cervical carcinoma at stage IB2-III, a clinical response rate ranging between 45% and 100% can be obtained following platinum-based chemotherapy *(table VIII)*. In our experience, a dramatic disease regression and symptomatic relief at the level of the primary tumour and vagina were observed in more than half of patients undergoing preoperative chemotherapy (substantial decrease or disappearance of vaginal bleeding and discharge), while a lower response was achieved in the parametria, bladder and lymph node (Benedetti Panici, personal experience). At the same time, we know that in pretreated patients with distant relapse of the disease, a clinical response to chemotherapy can be obtained in about one-third of the cases [27]. It is likely that a similar pattern of response can be achieved for newly-diagnosed stage IVB patients, despite the fact that the lower chemosensitivity of these tumours (due to a more aggressive biology of the disease) cannot be excluded.

Given the equivalence in survival between single and multiple agent chemotherapy [28], the frequent co-morbidities (obstructive uropathy, anaemia, etc.), and the importance of quality-of-life issues in this clinical setting, a platinum-based monochemotherapy (carboplatin AUC 4, cisplatin 50-75 mg/mq), until progression of the disease seems to be the most rational choice. The importance of supportive treatment (pain therapy, percutaneous urinary diversion, blood transfusions, hydro-electrolyte imbalance correction, psychological support, etc.) should never be overlooked when treating these incurable patients.

References

[1] Benedet J, Odicino F, Maisonneuve P, Severi G, Creasman W, Shephed J et al. Annual report on the results of treatment in gynaecological cancer. Carcinoma of the cervix uteri. *J Epidemiol Biostat* 1998 ; 3 : 5-34

[2] Benedetti Panici P, Greggi S, Scambia G, Amoroso M, Salerno MG, Maneschi F et al. Long-term survival following neoadjuvant chemotherapy and radical surgery in locally-advanced cervical cancer. *Eur J Cancer* 1998 ; 3 : 341-346

[3] Benedetti Panici P, Landoni F, Greggi S, Colombo A, Scambia G, Smaniotto D et al. Neoadjuvant chemotherapy and radical surgery vs exclusive radiotherapy in locally-advanced squamous cell cervical cancer. Results from the Italian multicenter randomized study. [abstract 1377]. *ASCO Proc* 1999 ; 18 : 357A

[4] Benedetti Panici P, Maneschi F, Cutillo G, Greggi S, Salerno MG, Amoroso M et al. Modified type IV-V radical hysterectomy with systematic pelvic and aortic lymphadenectomy in the treatment of patients with stage III cervical carcinoma. Feasibility, technique and clinical results. *Cancer* 1996 ; 78 : 2359-2365

[5] Benedetti Panici P, Maneschi F, Cutillo G, Congiu M, Franchi M, Amoroso M et al. Laparoscopic abdominal staging in locally-advanced cervical cancer. *Int J Gynecol Cancer* 1999 ; 9 : 194-197

[6] Benedetti Panici P, Scambia G, Baiocchi G, Greggi S, Mancuso S. Technique and feasibility of radical para-aortic and pelvic lymphadenectomy for gynecologic malignancies: a prospective study. *Int J Gynecol Cancer* 1991 ; 1 : 133-140

[7] Benedetti Panici P, Scambia G, Baiocchi G, Greggi S, Ragusa G, Gallo A et al. Neoadjuvant chemotherapy and radical surgery in locally-advanced cervical cancer. Prognostic factors for response and survival. *Cancer* 1991 ; 67 : 372-379

[8] Benedetti Panici P, Scambia G, Baiocchi G, Maneschi F, Greggi S, Mancuso S. Radical hysterectomy: a randomized study comparing two techniques for resection of the cardinal ligament. *Gynecol Oncol* 1993 ; 50 : 226-231

[9] Cosin JA, Fowler JM, Chen MD, Paley PJ, Carson LF, Twiggs LB. Pretreatment surgical staging of patients with cervical carcinoma: the case for lymph node debulking. *Cancer* 1998 ; 82 : 2241-2248

[10] Dottino PR, Plaxe SC, Beddo EA, Johnston C, Cohen CJ. Induction chemotherapy followed by radical surgery in cervical cancer. *Gynecol Oncol* 1991 ; 40 : 7-11

[11] Eifel PJ, Thoms WW, Smith TL, Morris M, Oswald MJ. The relationship between brachytherapy dose and otcome in patients with bulky endocervical tumors treated with radiation alone. *Int J Radiat Oncol Biol Phys* 1994 ; 28 : 113-118

[12] Fyles A, Keane TJ, Barton M, Simm J. The effect of treatment duration in the local control of cervix cancer. *Radiother Oncol* 1992 ; 25 : 273-279

[13] Girinsky T, Rey A, Roche B, Haie C, Gerbaulet A, Randrianarivello H et al. Overall treatment time in advanced cervical carcinomas. A critical parameter in treatment outcome. *Int J Radiat Oncol Biol Phys* 1993 ; 27 : 1051-1056

[14] Greer BE, Koh W, Figge D, Russel A, Cain J, Tamimi H. Gynecologic radiotherapy fields defined by intraoperative mesaurements. *Gynecol Oncol* 1990 ; 38 : 421-424

[15] Greer BE, Koh WJ, Stelzer KJ, Goff BA, Comsia N, Tran A. Expanded pelvic radiotherapy fields for treatment of local-regionally advanced carcinoma of the cervix: outcome and complications. *Am J Obstet Gynecol* 1996 ; 174 : 1141-1150

[16] Greggi S, Benedetti Panici P, Amoroso M, Scambia G, Paratore MP, Salerno MG et al. Intraperitoneal tumor spread in locally-advanced cervical carcinoma undergoing neoadjuvant chemotherapy. *Int J Gynecol Cancer* 1998 ; 8 : 207-214

[17] Hoskins WJ, Ford JH, Lutz MH, Averette HE. Radical hysterectomy and pelvic lymphadenectomy for the management of early invasive cancer of the cervix. *Gynecol Oncol* 1976 ; 4 : 278-290

[18] Hreshchyshyn MM, Aron BS, Boronow RC, Franklin EW 3rd, Shingleton HM. Hydroxyurea or placebo combined with radiation to treat stage IIIB and IV cervical cancer confined to the pelvis. *Int J Radiat Oncol Biol Phys* 1979 ; 5 : 317-322

[19] Keys H, Gibbon SK. Optimal management of locally-advanced cervical carcinoma. *J Natl Cancer Inst Monogr* 1996 ; 21 : 89-92

[20] Keys HM, Bundy BN, Stehman FB, Muderspech LI, Chofe WE, Suggs CL et al. Cisplatin, radiation, and adjuvant hysterectomy compared with radiation and adjuvant hysterectomy for bulky stage IB cervical carcinoma. *N Engl J Med* 1999 ; 340 : 1154-1161

[21] Kim RY, McGinnis LS, Spencer SA, Meredith RF, Jennelle RL, Salter MM. Conventional four-field pelvic radiotherapy technique without computed tomography-treatment planning in cancer of the cervix: potential geographic miss and its impact on pelvic control. *Int J Radiat Oncol Biol Phys* 1995 ; 31 : 109-112

[22] Komaki R, Brickner TJ, Hanlon AL, Owen JB, Hanks GE. Long-term results of treatment of cervical carcinoma in the United States in 1973, 1978, and 1983: patterns of care study (PCS). *Int J Radiat Oncol Biol Phys* 1995 ; 31 : 973-982

[23] Lanciano RM, Pajak TF, Martz K, Hanks GE. The influence of treatment time in outcome for squamous cell cancer of the uterine cervix treated with radiation: a patterns-of-care study. *Int J Radiat Oncol Biol Phys* 1992 ; 25 : 391-397

[24] Longsdon MD, Eifel PJ. FIGO IIIB squamous cell carcinoma of the cervix: an analysis of prognostic factors emphasizing the balance between external beam and intracavitary radiation therapy. *Int J Radiat Oncol Biol Phys* 1999 ; 43 : 763-775

[25] Morris M, Eifel PJ, Lu J, Grigsby PW, Levenback C, Stevens RE et al. Pelvic radiation with concurrent chemotherapy compared with pelvic and para-aortic radiation for high-risk cervical cancer. *N Engl J Med* 1999 ; 340 : 1137-1143

[26] Nag S, Orton C, Young D, Erickson B. The American Brachitherapy Society survey of brachitherapy practice for carcinoma of the cervix in the United States. *Gynecol Oncol* 1999 ; 73 : 111-118

[27] Omura GA. Chemotherapy for stage IVB or recurrent cancer of the uterine cervix. *J Natl Cancer Inst Mon* 1996 ; 21 : 123-126

[28] Omura GA, Blessing JA, Vaccarello L, Berman ML, Clarke-Pearson DL, Mutch DG et al. Randomized trial of cisplatin versus cisplatin + mitolactol versus cisplatin + ifosfamide in advanced squamous carcinoma of the cervix. A Gynecologic Oncology Group study. *J Clin Oncol* 1997 ; 15 : 165-171

[29] Parkin DM, Pisani P, Ferlay J. Global cancer statistics. *CA Cancer J Clin* 1999 ; 49 : 33-64

[30] Pedersen D, Bentzen SM, Overgaard J. Early and late radiotherapeutic morbidity in 442 consecutive patients with locally-advanced carcinoma of the uterine cervix. *Int J Radiat Oncol Biol Phys* 1994 ; 29 : 941-952

[31] Pedersen D, Bentzen SM, Overgaard J. Continuous or split-course combined external and intracavitary radiotherapy of locally-advanced carcinoma of the uterine cervix. *Acta Oncol* 1994 ; 33 : 547-555

[32] Pendlebury SC, Cahill S, Crandon AJ, Bull CA. Role of bipedal lymphangiogram in radiation treatment planning for cervix cancer. *Int J Radiat Oncol Biol Phys* 1993 ; 27 : 959-962

[33] Perez C, Kao M. Radiation therapy alone or continued with surgery in the treatment of barrel-shaped carcinoma of the uterine cervix (stages IB, IIA, IIB). *Int J Radiat Oncol Biol Phys* 1985 ; 11 : 1903-1909

[34] Petereit D, Sarkaria J, Chappel R, Fowler J, Hartmann T, Kinsella T et al. The adverse effect of treatment prolongation in cervical carcinoma. *Int J Radiat Oncol Biol Phys* 1995 ; 32 : 1301-1307

[35] Potish RA, Twiggs LB. On the lack of demonstrated clinical benefit of neoadjuvant cisplatinum therapy for cervical cancer. *Int J Radiat Oncol Biol Phys* 1999 ; 27 : 975-979

[36] Rose PG, Bundy BN, Watkins EB, Thigpen JT, Deppe G, Maiman MA et al. Concurrent cisplatin-based radiotherapy and chemotherapy for locally-advanced cervical cancer. *N Engl J Med* 1999 ; 340 : 1144-1153

[37] Rotman M, Pajak TF, Choi K, Clery M, Marcial V, Grigsby PW et al. Prophylactic extended-field irradiation of para-aortic lymph nodes in stages IIB and bulky IB and IIA cervical carcinomas. Ten-year treatment results of RTOG 79-20. *JAMA* 1995 ; 274 : 387-393

[38] Russell AH. Integration of diagnostic imaging in the clinical management of cervical cancer. *J Natl Cancer Inst Monogr* 1996 ; 21 : 35-41

[39] Russell AH, Walker JP, Anderson HW, Zukowski CL. Sagittal magnetic resonance imaging in the design of lateral radiation treatment portals for patients with locally-advanced squamous cancer of the cervix. *Int J Radiat Oncol Biol Phys* 1992 ; 23 : 449-455

[40] Sardi J, Giaroli A, Sananes C, Rueda NG, Vighi S, Ferreira M et al. Randomized trial with neoadjuvant chemotherapy in stage IIIB squamous carcinoma cervix uteri: an unexpected therapeutic management. *Int J Gynecol Cancer* 1996 ; 6 : 85-93

[41] Sardi J, Sananes C, Giarol A, Bermudez A, Ferreira MH, Soderini AH et al. Neoadjuvant chemotherapy in cervical carcinoma stage IIB: a randomized controlled trial. *Int J Gynecol Cancer* 1998 ; 8 : 441-450

[42] Sardi J, Sananes C, Giaroli A, Maya G, Di Paola G. Neoadjuvant chemotherapy in locally-advanced carcinoma of the cervix uteri. *Gynecol Oncol* 1990 ; 38 : 486-493

[43] Souhami L, Gil RA, Allan SE, Canary PCV, Araujo CMM, Pinto LHJ. Detrimental effect of neoadjuvant chemotherapy in patients with stage IIIB carcinoma of the cervix: results of a randomized trial. *Int J Oncol* 1992 ; 1 : 289-292

[44] Spanos WR Jr, Clery M, Perez CA, Grigsby PW, Doggett RL, Poulter CA et al. Late effect of multiple daily fraction palliation schedule for advanced pelvic malignancies (RTOG 8502). *Int J Radiat Oncol Biol Phys* 1994 ; 29 : 961-967

[45] Spanos WR Jr, Pajak TJ, Emami B,, Cooper JS, Russell AH, Cox JD. Radiation palliation of cervical cancer. *J Natl Cancer Inst Monogr* 1996 ; 21 : 127-130

[46] Spanos WR Jr, Wasserman T, Meoz R, Sala J, Kong J, Stetz J. Palliation of advanced pelvic malignant disease with large fraction pelvic irradiation and misonidazole: final report of RTOG phase I/II study. *Int J Radiat Oncol Biol Phys* 1987 ; 13 : 1479-1482

[47] Tattersall MH, Lorvidhaya V, Vootiprux V, Cheirsilpa A, Wong F, Azhar T et al. Randomized trial of epirubicin and cisplatin chemotherapy followed by pelvic radiation in locally-advanced cervical cancer: Cervical cancer study group of the Asian Oceanian Clinical Oncology Association. *J Clin Oncol* 1995 ; 13 : 444-451

[48] Van Nagell JR, Higgins RV. Clinical invasive carcinoma of the cervix: clinical features, diagnosis, staging and pre-treatment evaluation. In : Coppleson M ed. Gynecologic oncology. London : Churchill Livingstone, 1992 : 663-671

[49] Whitney CW, Sause W, Bundy BN, Malfetan JH, Hannigan EV, Fowler WC et al. Randomized comparison of fluorouracil plus cisplatin versus hydroxyurea as an adjunct to radiation therapy in stage IIB-IVA carcinoma of the cervix with negative para-aortic lymph nodes: a Gynecologic Oncology Group and Southwest Oncology Group study. *J Clin Oncol* 1999 ; 17 : 1339-1348

Chapter 13

Recurrence of cervical carcinoma: risk factors and treatment

Stelios Fotiou, Alexandros Rodolakis

S Fotiou, Professor, M.D., Ph.D.
A Rodolakis, M.D.
Dept. of Gynaecology, Saint Savas Oncological Hospital, 171 Alexandras Avenue, 11522 Athens, Greece.

Recurrence of cervical carcinoma: risk factors and treatment

S Fotiou, A Rodolakis

Abstract. — *Factors predicting the risk of recurrence in cervical carcinoma include clinical stage, volume of disease, lymphatic spread and possibly, adenomatous histology. In surgically treated early stages (I-IIa), positive nodes and surgical margins are strong predictors of recurrence. In node and margin negative patients, large tumours, deep stromal invasion and vascular space involvement correlate strongly to the risk of relapse. Management is difficult and depends mainly on the location of recurrence and previous treatment. Central pelvic recurrences have a better chance of cure. Following primary surgery, full radiation therapy should be instituted. Patients already radiated are candidates for aggressive surgery, usually in the form of exenteration. Recurrence involving the pelvic side-wall in patients not previously radiated is better treated with concurrent chemo-radiation. In already radiated patients, a combination of aggressive surgery and radiation may salvage selected patients. Extrapelvic metastases or pelvic disease after locoregional treatment is amenable to palliative chemotherapy only.*

Keywords: recurrent cervical cancer, risk factors, management.

Introduction

It is estimated that approximately one-third of patients with invasive cervical carcinoma will experience a relapse in the disease after initial treatment. In many studies, the form of the relapse, persistent or recurrent disease, is not clear. Recurrent cancer of the cervix can be defined as the regrowth of a tumour mass following treatment procedures that have removed all clinical evidence of gross disease. At least 3 months should elapse from primary healing obtained by radiotherapy or complete remission after successful surgery, before defining a regrowth as a tumour recurrence.

It has been shown that 55%-65% of cervical cancer recurrences will be diagnosed during the first year and 75%-80% within two years following the completion of primary treatment.

Several prognostic factors have been established as affecting the treatment outcome and increasing the risk of recurrence. Some of them are related to the tumour (clinical stage, tumour size and volume, histopathological characteristics of the disease) and others to the host (age, performance status), or to the treatment applied.

Risk factors

■ The FIGO stage

The clinical stage of disease affects survival and it has been shown that there is an increasing failure rate after primary treatment as stages advance. Patients treated with radiation alone were found to have an overall incidence of pelvic and distant recurrence that increased from 9.6% and 17.5% in stage Ib, to 41% and 42% respectively in stage III cases [16]. For early stage patients treated with surgery, with or without adjuvant radiotherapy, the reported incidence of recurrence also increases from about 10% for stage Ib to 20% for stage IIa cases [2].

■ Tumour size and volume of the disease

Tumours larger than 4 cm in diameter have a poorer prognosis compared to smaller tumours in comparably staged patients. The adverse effect on survival of increasing tumour size seems to be independent of the mode of primary treatment. Bulky, barrel-shaped tumours treated with radiation have a poorer prognosis, being associated with a higher rate of central treatment failures and a propensity to spreading in extrapelvic sites. The size of the primary tumour has a greater effect on survival in early (Ib-IIa) stage patients as compared to more advanced stage (IIb-III) disease. In the latter, volume and bilaterality are also important predictors of disease-free survival (DFS) [16].

■ Histological type and differentiation

The majority of patients with recurrent disease have squamous cell carcinoma of the cervix, but 10%-20% will exhibit other histology, principally adenocarcinoma. Although primary treatment is usually independent of the histological type of cancer, adenocarcinomas and adenosquamous carcinomas have been reported to recur more often after surgery, especially in distant sites. However, this propensity for an increasing risk of recurrence with adenomatous histology is not generally accepted. Some of the more rare histological types of cervical cancer such as clear cell, papillary serous and small cell carcinomas do show an increase in recurrence rates, but account for only a small fraction of all cervical cancers [20]. Poorly-differentiated tumours are considered to have a higher risk of recurrence, although this view is debated [27].

In patients treated with primary surgery (radical hysterectomy plus bilateral pelvic lymphadenectomy), additional risk factors for recurrence have been identified. Nodal involvement has been reported as a significant predictor of relapse. Node-positive patients are more likely to recur and within a shorter time than those with negative lymph nodes. Moreover, an increasing number of involved nodes, bilateralism, size of nodal metastases and para-aortic node involvement have been implicated as predictors of DFS [4, 24]. Patients with positive surgical margins also constitute a high-risk group for recurrence. In the series of Burke et al [1], 34.2% of stage Ib cases with positive nodes or excision margins recurred, in spite of postoperative radiation treatment. Both positive pelvic nodes and surgical margins have been proven to be independent variables, predictive of recurrence [2].

The depth of stromal invasion and vascular space involvement (VSI), two histologically-defined and reproducible parameters, have been related to the probability of lymph node metastasis and risk of relapse. Both these factors have been found to correlate strongly and independently to DFS in early stage, node-negative patients [4].

■ Risk groups

The reported recurrence rate in the early stages of cervical carcinoma (Ib-IIa) ranges between 10%-20%, while for the advanced stages (IIb-IVa), the rate increases to 20%-40%. The actual recurrence rate in advanced disease is due to an increasing number of patients with persistent disease. Thus, the early or advanced clinical stage of disease indicates a low-and a high-risk group of patients. Among patients with early stage disease, those found to have positive nodes or surgical margins following surgery constitute a group with a well-documented, increased risk for recurrence and the tumour recurs in 30%-50% of cases. Node and margin-negative patients, although they represent the lower-risk group in surgically-treated cases, account for nearly 50% of disease relapses for which identification of risk factors seems to be more difficult but equally important. Patients in this category who have large tumours (> 4 cm), deep cervical penetration or microscopic involvement of vascular spaces are considered at intermediate risk for disease recurrence. (Probability of recurrence at 3 years is from 2% to 31%) [4].

■ Primary treatment and risk of recurrence

Early stage disease can be treated with either surgery or radiation with comparable results; radiation therapy is applicable in all stages. In general, radical surgery is more frequently performed on young women who are in good physical condition. Patients selected for primary radiation treatment more often belong to an older age group, possibly with lower performance status and increased tumour aggressiveness. Young age has been associated with a more favourable prognosis in early stage disease, while a poorer survival rate has been reported in young women with advanced primary or recurrent disease [2, 18].

In surgically treated patients, it is mandatory to remove not only the central tumour with good margins but also any foci of malignant cells that may be entrapped in the distant parametria, even in the absence of metastatic disease in the pelvic nodes. For this purpose, extirpation of most of the uterosacral and cardinal ligaments has been advocated. However, this extensive class III radical hysterectomy entails an increased risk of serious post-operative morbidity and the extent of radical surgery should be tailored to the individual risk factors in each case. This approach will eliminate the risk of recurrence without unnecessarily compromising the patients' quality of life [6].

In patients treated with radiation, either primary or post-operative, the disease-free interval has been reported to be longer compared to that of patients treated by surgery alone. However, these differences can be attributed to different patient selection. The efficacy of radiation treatment can be affected by different local and systemic conditions, for example, the microvascularity of the tumour, chronic anaemia, etc. The dose of radiation delivered has also been correlated to treatment results. A higher incidence of pelvic recurrence has been reported in patients receiving doses lower than 50 Gy to the lateral parametrium [16]. Traditionally, patients with increased risk for recurrence have been treated with radiation alone (advanced stages) or with adjuvant radiation after surgery (early stages). Recent evidence based on the results of prospective randomised trials suggests that cisplatin-based chemotherapy administered concurrently with radiation can decrease the incidence of recurrence in patients with advanced stage disease and in high-risk surgically treated patients as well [15]. In patients with an intermediate risk of recurrence (node negative but with large tumours, deep stromal invasion and VSI), post-operative adjuvant radiation has been shown to decrease the recurrence rate significantly [19]. However, a longer follow-up is required to determine the impact of radiation therapy on the survival of these patients.

Pattern of recurrence

The majority of cervical cancer recurrences occurring after surgical treatment are located within the pelvis (60%-70%), involving only the area of the cervix and the vaginal apex (central recurrence), or the pelvic side-wall (lateral recurrence). Extrapelvic (distant) relapses account for about 1/3 of recurrences and appear more often in the lung or the abdomen. Following radiation therapy for early stage disease, the pattern of failure is different and recurrence is more often distant (76%) than pelvic (24%) [22].

High-risk tumours (advanced stage, positive nodes, adenomatous histology) recur more frequently in extrapelvic sites or on the pelvic side-wall. Relapses of low-risk, non-bulky tumours more often appear centrally in the pelvis and have a higher chance of cure. However, the possibility of disseminated disease (both pelvic and distant), even in patients presenting with an apparently localised recurrence, is high.

Surveillance of patients and diagnosis of recurrence

Since most recurrences (75%-80%) are diagnosed within the first two years post-treatment, frequent (every three months) patient evaluation during this period seems to be mandatory. Traditionally, clinical and cytological examinations are performed at every visit. Bimanual rectovaginal examination of the pelvis and physical evaluation of the abdominal, inguinal and supraclavicular areas are necessary. The assessment of the patient's physical condition is of great importance for the identification of clinical signs of disease relapse. The ominous presence of the triad: weight loss - leg oedema - pelvic pain - is highly suggestive of disease recurrence. Vaginal bleeding, the presence of a serosanguineous vaginal discharge or ureteral obstruction are symptoms or signs suggestive of relapse in the pelvic area. Pulmonary metastasis represents the most common distant site recurrence while bony metastases are relatively rare. Approximately 1/3 of cervical cancer recurrences are diagnosed at an asymptomatic stage. In most cases, diagnosis will be made by means of combined, conventional physical and gynaecological examinations and vaginal cytology [12]. However, the value of routine cytology has been debated, since smears suggestive of recurrence can be expected in nearly 60% of central pelvic recurrences only [2]. The routine use of chest X-rays, intravenous pyelogram or ultrasound of the kidneys in asymptomatic patients is not considered worthwhile, since they rarely increase the chances of cure. Nor should the newer imaging techniques, for example CT or MRI, be used for routine surveillance, but only when indicated by the patient's symptoms or clinical findings. The histological confirmation of recurrence is mandatory. In distant site metastasis, X-rays, bone or CT scans and MRI may be useful, while directed needle biopsies can establish the diagnosis. In the case of suspected central pelvic failure, scraping of the vaginal apex or endocervical curettage should be carried out. Lateral pelvic recurrence can be difficult to diagnose, especially in the presence of fibrotic, indurated parametria. Needle biopsies and aspiration cytology may provide an answer in these instances. At times, an exploratory diagnostic laparotomy becomes necessary.

Treatment

Recurrent carcinoma of the cervix is a discouraging clinical entity with a survival rate lower than 20%. Secondary treatment may prolong survival and eventually cure a small percentage of patients, whereas non-treated patients, as a rule, die of the disease. Management is often difficult and the chances of cure depend mainly on the site of the recurrence and on primary treatment. The evidence suggests that extrapelvic disease has a very low likelihood of cure, being suitable for palliative management only. For pelvic recurrences following primary surgical treatment, radiation therapy should be considered. Patients already treated with radiation should be evaluated for surgical intervention. At times, combined multimodal approaches should be taken into consideration.

■ Radiation therapy

Radiation treatment with curative intent is principally addressed to previously unradiated patients with recurrent cervical carcinoma confined to the pelvis. Whole pelvic external beam radiation plus intracavitary brachytherapy, with or without chemotherapy, is considered as standard treatment. This approach can lead to DFS rates of 20%-50% and local control rates of 20%-60%, depending on a number of factors but mainly on the location of the recurrence [11]. Patients with only central pelvic disease exhibit significantly higher survival rates as compared to those with recurrence extending to the pelvic side wall [10].

The large size of tumours in recurrence has been found to adversely affect the chances of local control. Early recurrence (within 6 months after primary treatment) is also reported to be associated with a higher mortality rate, possibly reflecting an increased biological aggressiveness of the tumour. The total radiation dose (at least 50 Gy) and the selection of the appropriate type of brachytherapy, i.e. ovoids, vaginal cylinder or interstitial implants, are also factors affecting prognosis [25].

The application of additional conventional radiation of the pelvis in previously radiated patients has been proven inadequate in controlling the disease. Re-irradiation with curative intent is only confined to those patients who had sub-optimal or incomplete primary radiation therapy. For small pelvic recurrences located within a fully-treated field, the use of multiple interstitial radiation sources through a perineal template has been suggested. In patients with late (over 5 years) vaginal recurrence with small-sized tumours, re-irradiation, mainly in the form of brachytherapy, can be applied with satisfactory results [26]. Finally, radiation therapy can be successfully applied for palliation and control of local disease outside the initial treatment field. Painful bone metastases or central nervous system lesions are specific indications.

■ Surgery

Following primary, or adjuvant post-operative radiation therapy, certain patients may develop recurrent disease treatable by surgery. Patients with central pelvic recurrence are the best candidates for radical operative procedures with curative intent. In the presence of lateral extension of the disease, the chances of curing the patient by surgery are greatly diminished. In case of a tumour mass fixed to the pelvic side-wall, very aggressive modalities combining ultraradical surgery and radiation therapy can be justified.

Radical hysterectomy and pelvic lymphadenectomy (RHPL)

In most centres, pelvic exenteration has become the standard treatment for central pelvic post-radiation recurrences. However, this operation still remains a formidable procedure. Therefore, RHPL has been suggested for the management of central tumours considered as resectable by less aggressive surgery. The reported cure rates after RHPL vary considerably. Rubin et al [17] combined the treatment results in 6 series and obtained an average 5 year survival figure of 62%. However, the application of RHPL in heavily radiated patients is associated with a high (30%-50%) rate of serious complications. On the other hand, comparison of survival rates after RHPL with data from exenteration series is not possible due to the different selection criteria. It seems that only carefully selected patients with small (less than 4 cm) recurrent tumours limited to the cervix and a normal preoperative intravenous pyelogram are likely to benefit from RHPL, especially in cases of poor surgical risk or refusal of exenteration [3, 13].

Pelvic exenteration

The procedure of pelvic exenteration was first described by Alex Brunswig in 1948. In spite of severe initial criticism, this operation is now established in many specialised, well organised centres. Procedure-related mortality has declined to less than 5% with an overall survival/cure rate of between 30% and 60% [14]. Pelvic exenteration is classified as anterior (removal of the bladder, vagina, cervix and uterus), posterior (removal of the rectum, vagina, cervix and uterus) or total exenteration, when the bladder and rectum are removed en bloc with the uterus, cervix, vagina and the pelvic floor. In selected patients a total exenteration may take place above the levator ani muscle (supralevator).

Pelvic examination plays a key role in the preoperative assessment of the patient. The presence of a small, central, mobile lesion is reassuring for the resectability of the disease. Patients with a tumour mass fixed to the pelvic side-wall should be eliminated from this procedure. Apart from the necessary histological confirmation of the recurrence, every effort should be made to exclude the possibility of an extrapelvic metastasis which is an absolute contraindication to exenteration. The careful assessment of the patient's general condition and mental state is mandatory. In this context, gross obesity, advanced age, systemic disease and psychological instability of the patient may affect the decision. The clinical triad of unilateral leg oedema, sciatic pain and ureteral obstruction is also considered pathognomonic of unresectable disease. In the case of operability remaining questionable, patients should be given the benefit of exploratory laparotomy and parametrial biopsies, because this can be their last hope for cure [5].

The final decision to carry out exenteration is taken during laparotomy. Meticulous exploration of the entire abdomen and the lower para-aortic nodes must exclude the presence of disease. The existence of positive pelvic nodes is an ominous prognostic sign which can lead to termination of the procedure although even in this group of patients, survivors have been reported after completion of the exenteration [14].

The description of the exenterative technique is beyond the scope of this chapter. It should, however, be emphasised that strenuous efforts have been made to decrease the permanent morbidity of the procedure by tailoring the extent of the operation to the individual patient's needs. In anterior exenteration, the bladder can only rarely be salvaged without compromising the patient's chances of cure. However, preservation of the rectosigmoid may occasionally be possible and at times a lower segmental resection and re-anastomosis of the bowel will be considered adequate. Although these modifications have been criticised for increasing the risk due to incomplete resection, they are important for the patient's quality of life.

The extenterative operation should be accompanied by procedures that reconstruct and rehabilitate the urinary and genital tracts as completely and functionally as possible. One of the greatest technical advances is the intestinal conduit for diversion of the urinary stream. The formation of a continent urinary pouch utilising a segment of bowel is the method currently employed; this allows the patient to go without an ileostomy bag and to use a catheter for self-catheterisation through a small umbilical stoma. If it has been decided preoperatively, the construction of a neovagina, using a split-thickness skin graft or an isolated segment of bowel, can be performed. Other surgeons have advocated the re-creation of the vaginal canal by using rectus abdominus or gracilis myocutaneous grafts. However, in many instances, patient concern about the maintenance of vaginal function after the operation is of low priority. Finally, in order to create a new pelvic floor, an omental graft is usually formed after mobilising the omentum from its attachments, preserving an adequate blood supply from the left gastroepiploic artery *(fig 1)*. This is placed in the pelvis to protect the denuded pelvic floor and can promote healing, help avoid bowel obstruction and reduce postoperative morbidity.

Major postoperative complications include pulmonary and cardiovascular catastrophes, sepsis, small bowel obstruction and fistula. Long-term morbidity is predominantly related to urinary complications (obstruction and infection).

■ Combined treatment

Recurrences of cervical carcinoma involving the pelvic side-wall represent a challenging therapeutic problem. These patients usually have failed treatment for a disease with ominous prognostic signs and are frequently radiated in the pelvis. Surgical or radiation therapy alone has historically given poor results in this form of recurrence for which chemotherapy has also proved disappointing. Selected patients with recurrent tumours infiltrating the lateral pelvic wall can be salvaged using combined treatment approaches.

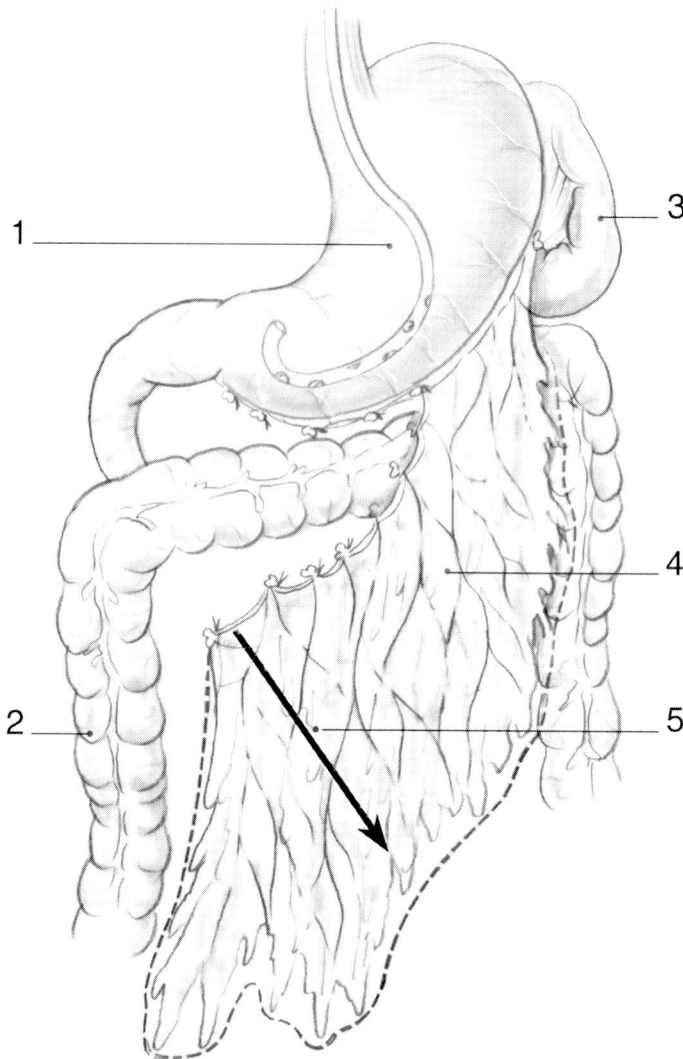

Figure 1. *Omental graft to cover the empty pelvis. 1. stomach; 2. ascending colon; 3. spleen; 4. omentum; 5. further incision to lengthen pedicle as appropriate. (Redrawn with permission from: Monaghan JM. The role of exenterative surgery. In: Heintz APM, Allen DG eds. Practical procedures for the gynaecological oncologist. Amsterdam: Elsevier, 1998: 87-95).*

Concurrent chemo-radiation

In patients not previously radiated, concurrent chemotherapy and radiation has been recommended as salvage therapy in the presence of recurrent pelvic disease, even extending to the lateral pelvic wall [23].

Intra-operative radiation therapy (IORT)

A combination of extensive surgical resection of a recurrent tumour involving the pelvic side-wall with intra-operative electron-beam radiation of the tumour bed has been proposed as salvage treatment. However, this approach is mainly addressed to patients not previously fully-radiated, since additional external radiation is required to achieve cancericidal doses [21].

Combined operative-radiation therapy (CORT)

The objective of this approach is to remove the tumour centrally, with good margins, and at the pelvic wall at least macroscopically, and to irradiate the tumour bed postoperatively by applying tube-guided brachytherapy. CORT is a multistep procedure consisting of surgical exploration, ablation, implantation of the guide-tubes in the tumour bed, pelvic wall plasty and reconstruction. Brachyterapy starts in the second postoperative week. Candidates for this treatment are patients with recurrent side-wall tumour not exceeding 5 cm in diameter, after prior pelvic radiation for primary or recurrent disease. The presence of extrapelvic metastases, bad general condition and advanced age are considered contraindications [8].

The laterally extended endopelvic resection (LEER) technique

This was developed by Hockel as an evolution of the surgical technique used in CORT [9]. With this approach, the exenterative procedure is extended laterally with the aim of completely removing the side-wall tumour en bloc with the parietal endopelvic fascia and the adjacent pelvic wall muscles and/or internal iliac vessels. The LEER technique is indicated for the treatment of infrailiac side-wall tumours not larger than 5 cm in diameter, recurring more than 5 months after primary treatment. Initial experience has shown that a 35% five year survival rate can be achieved, while the overall complication rate does not exceed 22%. When lateral surgical margins are free of disease, which can be achieved in about 1/3 of cases, the postoperative tube-guided brachytherapy can be avoided.

■ Palliative treatment

Despite the contribution of screening programmes to early diagnosis and the improvement of treatment modalities, approximately 1/3 of the patients with cervical cancer finally die of the disease. Patients with extrapelvic metastasis or pelvic disease after locoregional therapy only depend on chemotherapy. Cisplatin has been proven to be the most effective drug in patients with squamous carcinoma of the cervix, especially in those who have not received prior chemotherapy. Since chemotherapy has not resulted in the cure of any patient with recurrent cervical cancer, either in the pelvis or distantly, cytotoxic treatment should only be administered for palliation, taking into consideration individual patient needs and prospects.

Recurrent pelvic disease can result in bilateral ureteral obstruction and uraemia. In patients initially treated by surgery and without evidence of distant site metastasis, transvesicle or percutaneous ureteral catheters should be placed and radiotherapy with curative intent should be instituted. When this is not possible, the creation of a urinary conduit before the commencement of treatment should be considered. Patients with bilateral, ureteral obstruction following a full dose of pelvic radiation therapy are beyond any curative treatment option. In these cases, using a stent or nephrostomy to overcome the obstruction can be a source of subsequent regret since no "useful life" can be achieved for these patients [7].

References

[1] Burke TW, Hoskins WJ, Heller BP, Bibro MC, Weiser EB, Park RC. Prognostic factors associated with radical hysterectomy failure. *Gynecol Oncol* 1987 ; 26 : 153-159

[2] Cary A, Free KE, Wright RG, Shield PW. Carcinoma of the cervix: recurrences in Queensland 1982-1986. *Int J Gynecol Cancer* 1992 ; 2 : 207-214

[3] Coleman RL, Keeney ED, Freedman RS, Burke TW, Eifel PJ, Rutledge FN. Radical hysterectomy for recurrent carcinoma of the uterine cervix after radiotherapy. *Gynecol Oncol* 1994 ; 55 : 29-35

[4] Delgado C, Bundy BN, Zaino R, Sevin BU, Creasman WT, Major F. Prospective surgical-pathological study of disease free interval in patients with stage Ib squamous cell carcinoma of the cervix: A GOG study. *Gynecol Oncol* 1990 ; 38 : 352-357

[5] Di Saia PJ, Creasman WT. Invasive cervical cancer. In : Di Saia PJ, Creasman WT eds. Clinical gynecologic oncology. St. Louis : CV Mosby, 1997 ; 51-106

[6] Fotiou S, Tserkezoglou A, Hatzieleftheriou G, Apostolikas N. Class III vs class II radical hysterectomy in stage Ib cervical carcinoma: a comparison of morbidity and survival. *Int J Gynecol Cancer* 1997 ; 7 : 117-121

[7] Grant PT. Urologic surgery for the gynaecologic oncologist. In : Heintz AP, Allen DG eds. Practical procedures for the gynaecological oncologist. Amsterdam : Elsevier, 1998 : 121-134

[8] Hockel M. Combined operative and radiotherapeutic treatment (CORT). In : Heintz AP, Allen DG eds. Practical procedures for the gynaecological oncologist. Amsterdam : Elsevier, 1998 : 247-266

[9] Hockel M. Laterally extended endopelvic resection: Surgical treatment of infrailiac pelvic wall recurrences of gynaecologic malignancies. *Am J Obstet Gynecol* 1999 ; 180 : 306-312

[10] Ijaz T, Eifel PJ, Burke T, Oswald MJ. Radiation therapy of pelvic recurrence after radical hysterectomy for cervical carcinoma. *Gynecol Oncol* 1998 ; 70 : 241-246

[11] Lanciano R. Radiotherapy for the treatment of locally recurrent cervical cancer. *J Natl Cancer Inst Monogr* 1996 ; 21 : 113-115

[12] Larson DM, Copeland LJ, Malone JM, Stringer CA, Gershenson DM, Edwards CL. Diagnosis of recurrent cervical carcinoma after radical hysterectomy. *Obtet Gynecol* 1988 ; 71 : 6-9

[13] Maneo A, Landoni F, Cormio G, Colombo A, Mangioni C. Radical hysterectomy for recurrent or persistent cervical cancer following radiation therapy. *Int J Gynecol Cancer* 1999 ; 9 : 295-301

[14] Monaghan JM. The role of exenterative surgery. In : Heintz AP, Allen DG eds. Practical procedures for the gynaecological oncologist. Amsterdam : Elsevier, 1998 : 87-95

[15] National Cancer Institute, Bethesda. Clinical announcement on cervical cancer: Chemotherapy plus radiation improves survival. Press Release, Feb. 22, 1999

[16] Perez CA, Grigsby PW, Nene SM, Camel HM, Galakatos A, Kao MS et al. Effect of tumour size on the prognosis of carcinoma of the uterine cervix treated with radiation alone. *Cancer* 1992 ; 69 : 2796-2806

[17] Rubin SC, Hoskins WJ, Lewis JL. Radical hysterectomy for recurrent cervical cancer following radiation therapy. *Gynecol Oncol* 1987 ; 27 : 316-322

[18] Rutledge FN, Michell MF, Munsell M, Bass S, Mac Guffee V, Atkinson FN. Youth as a prognostic factor in carcinoma of the cervix: A matched analysis. *Gynecol Oncol* 1992 ; 44 : 123-130

[19] Sedlis A, Bundy BN, Rotman MZ, Lentz SS, Muderspash LI, Zaino RJ. A randomized trial of pelvic radiation therapy versus no further therapy in selected patients with stage Ib carcinoma of the cervix after radical hysterectomy and pelvic lymphadenectomy: A gynecologic oncology group study. *Gynecol Oncol* 1999 ; 73 : 177-183

[20] Shingleton HM, Bell MC, Fremgen A, Chmiel JS, Russell AH, Jones WB et al. Is there really a difference in survival of women with squamous cell carcinoma adenocarcinoma and adenosquamous cell carcinoma of the cervix ? *Cancer* 1995 ; 76 (suppl 10) : 1948-1955

[21] Stelzer KJ, Koh WJ, Greer BE, Cain JM, Tamini HK, Figge DC et al. The use of intraoperative radiation therapy in radical salvage for recurrent cervical cancer: outcome and toxicity. *Am J Obstet Gynecol* 1995 ; 172 : 1881-1888

[22] Thomas GM, Dembo AJ. Is there a role for adjuvant pelvic radiotherapy after radical hysterectomy in early stage cervical cancer ? *Int J Gynecol Cancer* 1991 ; 1 : 1-8

[23] Thomas GM, Dembo AJ, Myhr T, Black B, Pringle JF, Rawlings G. Long-term results of concurrent radiation and chemotherapy for carcinoma of the cervix recurrent after surgery. *Int J Gynecol Cancer* 1993 ; 3 : 193-198

[24] Tinga DJ, Bouma J, Boonstra H, Aalders JG. Symptomatology, localization and treatment of recurrent cervical carcinoma. *Int J Gynecol Cancer* 1992 ; 2 : 179-188

[25] Virostek LJ, Kim RY, Spencer SA, Meredith RF, Jenelle RLS, Soong SJ et al. Postsurgical recurrent carcinoma of the cervix: reassessment and results of radiation therapy options: *Radiology* 1996 ; 201 : 559-563

[26] Xiang EW, Shu-Mo C, Ya-Quin D, Ke W. Treatment of late recurrent vaginal malignancy after initial radiotherapy for carcinoma of the cervix: an analysis of 73 cases: *Gynecol Oncol* 1998 ; 69 : 125-129

[27] Zaino RJ, Ward S, Delgado G, Bundy B, Gore H, Fetter G et al. Histopathologic predictors of the behavior of surgically treated stage Ib squamous cell carcinoma of the cervix: *Cancer* 1992 ; 69 : 1750-1758

Chapter 14

Management of early cervical carcinoma associated with pregnancy

Jordi Xercavins, Antonio Gil-Moreno

J Xercavins, Professor of Obstetrics and Gynaecology.
A Gil-Moreno, Unit of Gynaecological Oncology.
Department of Obstetrics and Gynaecology, Hospital Universitario Materno-Infantil Vall d'Hebron, Autonomous University of Barcelona, Barcelona, Spain.

Management of early cervical carcinoma associated with pregnancy

J Xercavins, A Gil-Moreno

Abstract. – *Invasive cervical cancer complicating pregnancy is rare. Pregnancy may provide an opportunity for patients not previously included in routine cervical cancer screening programmes to be diagnosed at earlier stages, when prenatal care includes routine Pap smear testing during the first trimester. Approximately 90% of cases present with early-stage disease, mostly in the absence of clinical symptoms at the time of diagnosis. Although treatment options should be based on FIGO clinical staging, gestational age and the patient's desires regarding the pregnancy, the therapeutic approach to cervical cancer is similar for pregnant women and their non-pregnant counterparts. Overall survival and disease-free survival rates based on the stage of the disease are comparable in pregnant and non-pregnant patients and are not influenced by the mode of delivery or treatment modalities including planned delay to await fetal maturity.*

Keywords: early cervical carcinoma, pregnancy, treatment delay, neoadjuvant chemotherapy.

Introduction

Invasive cervical cancer complicating pregnancy is relatively rare. The reported incidence varies, depending or not on the inclusion of postpartum patients, although strictly speaking only patients diagnosed with invasive cervical cancer during pregnancy should be considered [14]. For this reason, only a few institutions would have followed a sufficient number of such cases to draw firm conclusions on how best to treat the malignancy and decide timing to initiate therapy. The influence of pregnancy on the behaviour of the tumour is largely unknown [12, 17]. The prognosis of early-stage cervical cancer is similar for pregnant and non-pregnant patients [17, 19]. There is a consensus in the literature defining "early cervical carcinoma" as an invasive carcinoma that is strictly confined to the cervix, or involves the vagina but not as far as the lower third, is no greater than 4 cm in diameter, and with no obvious parametrial involvement or spread of the growth to adjacent or distant organs [19, 30, 37]. This corresponds to stages IA1, IA2, IB1 and IIA (not bulky) of the International Federation of Gynaecology and Obstetrics (FIGO) staging of carcinoma of the cervix [7]. In contrast, bulky stage IB2 and IIA cervical cancers exceed 4 cm in diameter, have a poorer survival, high lymph node involvement and a higher recurrence rate.

Epidemiology

Carcinoma of the cervix represents approximately 20% of all gynaecological cancers, which in turn constitute one-fifth of all malignancies in women. According to a review of the literature [26], human papilloma virus (HPV) DNA has been identified in 20% to 100% of cervical carcinomas, depending on the method used to detect infection by HPV.

Invasive carcinoma of the cervix is reported to occur once in approximately every 2,000–10,000 pregnancies [10] and the combination of pregnancy and cervical cancer is rare: 1%–3% of cervical cancers are diagnosed during pregnancy [12, 19, 37]. The age of the patients varies between 19 and 46 years, with a mean age of 31–34 years (about 14–16 years younger than that of non-pregnant women). Between 80% and 90% of cervical carcinomas are squamous, although in recent years an increasing number of patients diagnosed with various subtypes of adenocarcinoma, such as villoglandular papillary adenocarcinoma, have been revealed [18, 38] *(fig 1)*. An increased risk of adenocarcinoma of the cervix associated with oral contraceptive use has been observed [36].

Diagnosis

For women not previously included in routine cervical cancer screening programmes, pregnancy may provide an opportunity to be diagnosed at earlier stages when prenatal care includes routine Pap smear testing during the first trimester of gestation. When the smear tests performed during pregnancy are indicative of cervical intraepithelial lesions, whatever the severity, colposcopy with guided biopsies are mandatory [11, 23]. Inadequate sampling and errors of interpretation of colposcopic images are the most common causes of false-negative results.

The cervix of pregnant women allows colposcopic evaluation since eversion of the columnar epithelium facilitates visualisation of the transformation zone as pregnancy

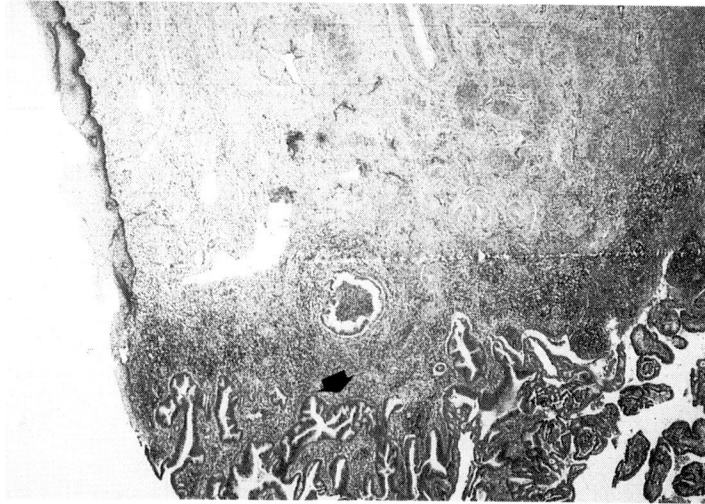

Figure 1. *Villoglandular papillary adenocarcinoma of the cervix: papillary projections and glands of regular size and morphology with scarce cytological atypia and abundant stroma (haematoxylin-eosin x 20).*

progresses. The sensitivity of colposcopy is higher than that of Pap smears with a false-negative rate lower than 10%. Colposcopy with directed punch biopsy or cervical conisation is used to diagnose an invasive malignancy. Conisation performed after 20 weeks of pregnancy leads to an extremely high rate of complications (20%–30%) [12, 23]. In a series of 180 cone biopsies during pregnancy, blood transfusion was required in 9% of cases due to operative blood loss [1]. Other complications included infection, cervical stenosis, cervical incompetence, postoperative phlebitis, pulmonary embolisation and chorioamnionitis. Foetal complications secondary to conisation were: spontaneous abortion, premature delivery, immature foetuses and sepsis [1, 12]. Although laser conisation and loop electrosurgical excision of the transformation zone produce suitable tissue specimens for histopathology, minimising the rate of complications with no foetal losses when these procedures are performed in the first trimester of pregnancy [4, 27], colposcopy-guided biopsy has replaced cervical cone biopsy, yielding an accurate diagnosis in 99.5% of cases, with a complication rate decreased to 0.6% [12]. Cervical cone biopsy is currently used when: colposcopic examination is unsuccessful; colposcopic findings are not consistent with the severity of cytological abnormalities; colposcopy or directed biopsy suggests a microinvasive carcinoma; or the guided biopsy shows an adenocarcinoma [6, 12, 13, 23, 27]. Other authors advocate minimal conisation to exclude stromal invasion [4]. Endocervical curettage during pregnancy should not be performed to avoid trauma within the endocervical canal [2].

Clinical staging according to the 1995 FIGO system should be performed by gynaecological oncologists and/or radiotherapists [30, 31]. In the rules for clinical staging, all patients should be evaluated with a detailed history and physical examination, paying particular attention to speculum inspection and palpation of the pelvic organs with bimanual and rectovaginal examinations to assess tumour size, extension into the vagina and parametrial involvement. Most pregnant patients with invasive carcinoma of the cervix have early-stage disease, despite the fact that many have large tumours and are diagnosed late in their pregnancy [19]. In addition to clinical staging, magnetic resonance imaging (MRI) is a valuable modality for determining tumour size, degree of

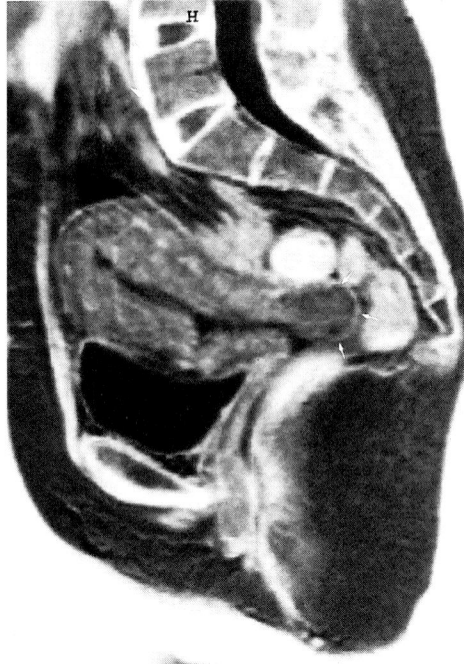

Figure 2. *Sagittal MRI scan showing a puerperal uterus, increased in size, and caesarean scar at the uterine segment. Cervical cancer, 3 x 2.5 cm in diameter, at the posterior lip.*

stromal penetration and parametrial extension, with a staging accuracy of 90% [34] *(fig 2)*. The first symptom of invasive cervical cancer is usually abnormal vaginal bleeding, often following coitus, although 20%–30% of patients may be asymptomatic. Therefore, vaginal bleeding during pregnancy should always be investigated.

Treatment

The treatment schema for patients with invasive cervical cancer in pregnancy varies with gestational age at diagnosis, FIGO stage and the patient's desires regarding the pregnancy. Treatment modalities directly interfere with maintenance of pregnancy and, not uncommonly, lead to difficult ethical, emotional and social decisions for the expectant parents and the physicians concerned. Data regarding the influence of pregnancy on the natural history of the tumour biology are inconclusive but negative effects on the prognosis of cervical cancer have not been demonstrated. Although treatment strategies are basically similar to that for non-pregnant women, the dilemma arises when patients present after the 20th or 24th week of pregnancy [8]. There should be a thorough discussion of the risks and options with both parents before any treatment is undertaken.

■ Treatment before 20 weeks of gestation

The therapeutic approach to cervical cancer diagnosed before 20 weeks gestation is similar for pregnant women and their non-pregnant counterparts. The standard treatment for early stages is radical hysterectomy and pelvic retroperitoneal or aorto-pelvic lymphadenectomy with ovarian conservation and/or external-beam irradiation and brachytherapy. Radiation resulted in spontaneous abortion during the first trimester of pregnancy in 70% of cases before 40 grays (Gy) were delivered [31]. External-beam radiation doses range from 40–60 Gy over an average of 34 days. Intracavitary therapy is administered using colpostats with either radium-226 or cesium-137 sources, with a mean dose to Point A of 55 Gy and to Point B of 20 Gy. In the few studies that have evaluated the radiotherapeutic management of cervical carcinoma diagnosed during pregnancy, no differences in short term toxicity and late complications from historical controls have been found [31].

▪ Treatment after 20 weeks of gestation

When patients present at the beginning of the third trimester of pregnancy, delay of treatment until the foetus has a better chance of survival may involve progression of the clinical stage of the disease. Materno-foetal survival is not affected by the mode of delivery (vaginal, caesarean section). Vaginal delivery may be allowed in the absence of large lesions that may cause infectious or haemorrhagic problems. Treatment-related complication rates are comparable in pregnant and non-pregnant patients, although with a greater amount of blood loss [31]. The softening of tissues in pregnancy gives the technical advantage of developing cleavage planes easily and with careful surgical technique, radical hysterectomy and pelvic lymphadenectomy are safe in pregnancy, with no differences in mean hospital stay, infection rates or ureterovesical dysfunction [24, 29, 30]. With the option of radiotherapy, similar results as with surgery are obtained, even better in the case of large tumours [31]. Modern neonatal intensive care units and prompt treatment of pulmonary maturity with steroids and surfactants can now dramatically influence decisions for delivery [16]. This should be taken into consideration when immediate treatment is planned in cases with obvious invasion and the possibility of a viable foetus [23].

Candidates for adjuvant radiotherapy would be: patients undergoing radical surgery with associated predictors of poor outcome, including lymph-vascular space invasion and lymph node metastasis; some histological subtypes, such as non-villoglandular adenocarcinoma; extensive stromal invasion with parametrial involvement and high-risk HPV infection [31].

▪ Treatment of stage IA1 disease

In these cases, the measured invasion of stroma is no greater than 3 mm in depth and no wider than 7 mm. The diagnosis is made on histological grounds and clinical staging is not altered by lymph-vascular space invasion. Cervical conisation may be a diagnostic and therapeutic procedure, especially if the margins of the cone are negative and there is no lymph-vascular space involvement [23, 37]. These patients may be followed to term and delivered vaginally. In the absence of histopathological factors of poor outcome, patients who have this conservative treatment - and if further childbearing is desired - must be followed closely with periodical cytology, colposcopy and endocervical curettage. In contrast, if further childbearing is not desired, vaginal hysterectomy or abdominal hysterectomy following caesarean section without pelvic lymph node dissection may be performed for the treatment of stage IA1 invasive cancer [15, 30] (*fig 3*).

▪ Treatment of stages IA2, IB1 and not bulky IIA disease

Patients with invasive cervical cancer diagnosed after 20 weeks gestation, mostly in the second and third trimesters, should be treated immediately with radical hysterectomy

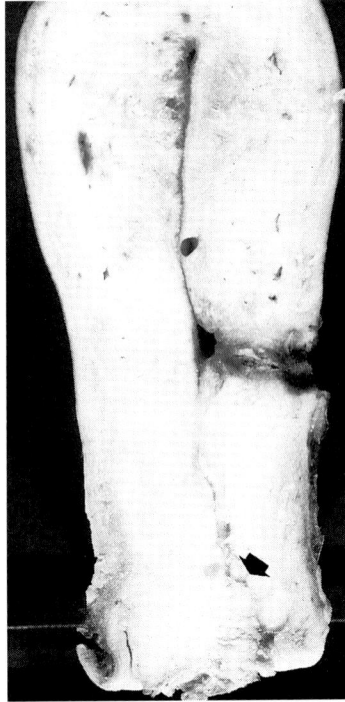

Figure 3. *Radical hysterectomy specimen in which a caesarean scar prior to definitive surgical treatment can be observed. Exophytic tumour with depth invasion up to 7 mm in the posterior cervical lip.*

and bilateral pelvic lymphadenectomy (stage IA2) or aorto-pelvic lymphadenectomy (stages IB1 and not bulky IIA) or with radiotherapy [30, 31]. During the first trimester of pregnancy, radical surgery is performed with the foetus *in situ*. For women in the second trimester of pregnancy, the recommended treatment is classical caesarean section, followed by radical hysterectomy and pelvic lymph node dissection [37]. Although primary radiation therapy is a safe treatment modality in the first and second trimesters, surgical treatment offers immediate termination in early pregnancy and avoids mental anguish and emotional suffering related to the expectation of spontaneous abortion or possible uterine evacuation associated with radiation therapy. Another possibility is to perform a hysterectomy followed by brachytherapy 2 weeks later.

Patients with FIGO stage I disease in whom invasive cervical cancer is diagnosed after 20 weeks may have their cancer treatment delayed to increase the likelihood of foetal maturity without compromising maternal prognosis [10, 30, 31, 32, 33, 35]. It is important to discuss the risks and options before planned delay in therapy is instituted. These patients must be strictly followed every 3–4 weeks to assess progression of the disease. Patients can also be effectively treated by either radical surgery or radiotherapy. Surgery has a clear advantage over radiotherapy for these young women, namely, the ability to preserve ovarian and sexual function [19, 22, 24, 40]. Most gynaecological oncologists recommend classic caesarean section followed immediately by radical hysterectomy and pelvic lymphadenectomy [24, 35, 37]. In high-risk patients, it is probably unwise to delay therapy [30]. It has been shown that in pregnant patients with early-stage disease, delayed therapy does not adversely effect survival [19].

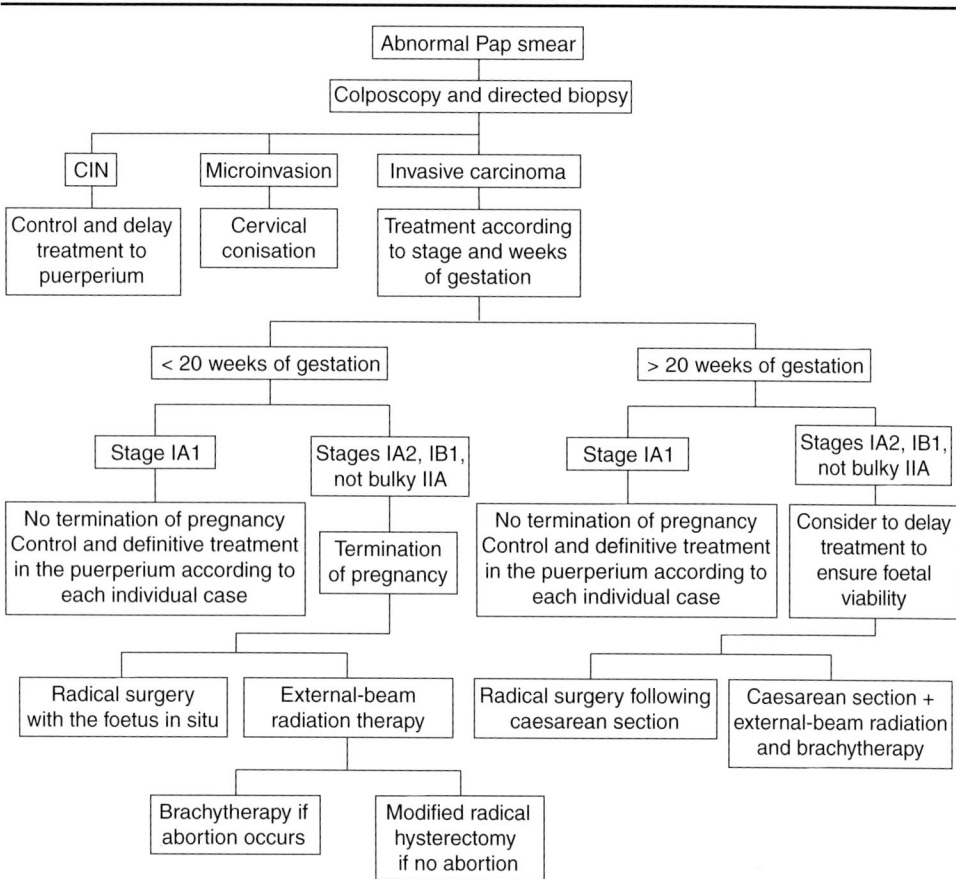

Figure 4. *Diagnostic and therapeutic approach of early invasive cervical carcinoma during pregnancy.*

Figure 4 shows diagnostic and therapeutic approaches to early cervical carcinoma during pregnancy.

■ Neoadjuvant chemotherapy

The results obtained in cervical cancer patients with neoadjuvant chemotherapy in combination with radiotherapy or surgery cannot be easily compared because studies are uncontrolled, the series are small, they often have short follow-up and the criteria for patient selection are not always clear [5, 21]. There has been one report of neoadjuvant chemotherapy in the treatment of locally advanced cervical carcinoma in two patients diagnosed early in the second trimester who strongly desired continuation of their pregnancies [35]. They were treated with 4–6 cycles of vincristine and cisplatin and experienced a dramatic reduction in tumour volume, rendering radical hysterectomy feasible at the time of caesarean section. Both patients tolerated chemotherapy well and there were no adverse foetal effects. An increased incidence of spontaneous abortions and major birth defects when various chemotherapeutic agents were used during embryogenesis in pregnant women with different malignancies has been reported [40], but such a risk was not demonstrable in pregnant women exposed to chemotherapy after the first trimester. Exposure to antineoplastic agents in the second and third trimesters of pregnancy may result in intrauterine growth retardation, premature birth, haematopoietic suppression, infertility, impaired mental development and second-generation carcinogenesis [9]. References to efficacy of neoadjuvant chemotherapy for patients diagnosed early in pregnancy were not found; however, if an expectant mother refuses to sacrifice her pregnancy, consideration should be made for this treatment modality in an effort to allow time to reach foetal viability by preventing progression of the disease.

■ Concurrent chemoradiation

The primary goal of combining radiation therapy with concurrent chemotherapy is to use chemotherapeutic agents to sensitise tumour cells to the effects of radiotherapy. Drugs most commonly given concurrently with radiation therapy include cisplatin, hydroxyurea, 5-fluorouracil and mitomycin-C. It has recently been shown that regimens of radiotherapy and chemotherapy that contain cisplatin improve the rates of survival and progression-free survival amongst non-pregnant women with locally advanced cervical cancer [20, 25, 28].

Survival

When pregnant and non-pregnant patients with invasive cervical carcinoma are matched by disease stage, both groups show similar overall survival rates and disease-free intervals [12, 19, 30, 31]. Overall outcome is not influenced by route of delivery (vaginal or caesarean section) [14, 37] or modality of treatment, including planned delay of therapy until foetal maturity is achieved [16, 23, 31, 37, 39]. When patients are stratified by age groups, differences in survival between younger and older groups are not found either [19]. Five year cumulative survival for patients with early-stage disease is 80%–90% [37], even including patients with planned delay in treatment [19]. The clinical stage of the disease is the most important determinant of prognosis. Survival may be worse for patients diagnosed in the third trimester or in the puerperium because the diagnosis of cancer tends to be associated with a more advanced clinical stage [3, 37].

Follow-up

Close follow-up conducted by gynaecological oncologists and radiotherapists from oncological units every 3 months during the first 2 years, every 4 months from the 3rd to the 5th year and at annual intervals thereafter seems advisable.

It should be noted that 90% of recurrences are detected at 2 years of treatment or earlier [31]. Control visits must include careful physical examination and Pap smear testing combined with biopsy when there is clinical, cytological or colposcopic suspicion of local tumour recurrence. Suspected spread to distant organs should be confirmed by computed tomography (CT) or MRI scans of the abdomen, bone scintigraphy or brain CT scan.

References

[1] Averette HE, Nasser N, SL, Little WA. Cervical conization in pregnancy. Analysis of 180 operations. *Am J Obstet Gynecol* 1970 ; 106 : 543-549

[2] Bakry YN, Akhtar M, Al-Amri A. Carcinoma of the cervix in a pregnant woman with negative Pap smears and colposcopic examination. *Acta Obstet Gynecol Scand* 1990 ; 69 : 657-658

[3] Baltzer J, Regenbrecht ME, Kopcke W, Zander J. Carcinoma of the cervix and pregnancy. *Int J Gynecol Obstet* 1990 ; 31 : 317-323

[4] Békássy Z. Laser miniconization procedure. *Int J Gynecol Obstet* 1996 ; 55 : 237-256

[5] Benedetti P, Scambia G, Baiocchi G, Greggi S, Ragusa G, Gallo A et al. Neoadjuvant chemotherapy and radical surgery in locally advanced cervical cancer: prognostic factors for response and survival. *Cancer* 1991 ; 67 : 372-379

[6] Connor JP. Non-invasive cervical cancer complicating pregnancy. *Obstet Gynecol Clin North Am* 1998 ; 25 : 331-342

[7] Creasman WT. New gynecologic cancer staging (editorial). *Gynecol Oncol* 1995 ; 58 : 157-158

[8] Creasman WT, Rutledge F, Fletcher G. Carcinoma of the cervix associated with pregnancy. *Obstet Gynecol* 1970 ; 36 : 495-499

[9] Doll DC, Ringenberg QS, Yarbro JW. Anti-neoplastic agents and pregnancy. *Semin Oncol* 1989 ; 16 : 337-346

[10] Duggan B, Muderspach LI, Roman LD, Curtin JP, D'Ablaing G 3rd, Morrow CP. Cervical cancer in pregnancy: reporting on planned delay therapy. *Obstet Gynecol* 1993 ; 82 : 598-602

[11] Giraud JR, Poulain P, Renaud-Giono A, Burtin F, Burtin JF, Proudhon JF et al. CIN and pregnancy. Apropos of 16 cases and review of the literature. *J Gynecol Obstet Biol Reprod* 1997 ; 26 : 496-502

[12] Hacker NF, Berek JS, Lagasse LD, Charles EH, Savage EV, Moore JG. Carcinoma of the cervix associated with pregnancy. *Obstet Gynecol* 1982 ; 59 : 735-746

[13] Hanningan EV, Witehouse HH, Atkinson WD, Becker SN. Cone biopsy during pregnancy. *Obstet Gynecol* 1982 ; 60 : 450-455

[14] Hempling RE. Cervical cancer. In : Piver MS ed. Handbook of gynecologic oncology. Boston : Little, Brown and Company, 1996 : 125-126

[15] Hoffman MS, Roberts WS, Fiorica JV, Angel JL, Finan MA, Cavanagh D. Elective cesarean hysterectomy for treatment of cervical neoplasia. An update. *J Reprod Med* 1993 ; 38 : 186-188

[16] Hopkins MP, Lavin JP. Cervical cancer in pregnancy (editorial). *Gynecol Oncol* 1996 ; 63 : 293

[17] Hopkins MP, Morley GW. The prognosis and management of cervical cancer associated with pregnancy. *Obstet Gynecol* 1992 ; 80 : 9-13

[18] Hurteau JA, Rodriguez GC, Kay HH, Bentley RC, Clarke-Pearson D. Villoglandular adenocarcinoma of the cervix: a case report. *Obstet Gynecol* 1995 ; 85 : 906-908

[19] Jones WB, Shingleton HM, Russell A, Fremgen AM, Clive RE, Winchester DP et al. Cervical carcinoma and pregnancy. A national patterns of care study of the American College of Surgeons. *Cancer* 1996 ; 77 : 1479-1488

[20] Keys HM, Bundy BN, Stehman FB, Muderspach LI, Chafe WE, Suggs CL 3rd et al. Cisplatin, radiation, and adjuvant hysterectomy compared with radiation and adjuvant hysterectomy for bulky stage IB cervical carcinoma. *N Engl J Med* 1999 ; 340 : 1154-1161

[21] Kim DS, Moon H, Kim KT, Hwuang W, Cho SH, Kim SR. Two-year survival: preoperative adjuvant chemotherapy in the treatment of cervical cancer stages IB and II with bulky tumor. *Gynecol Oncol* 1989 ; 33 : 225-230

[22] Lewandowski GS, Vaccarello L, Copeland LJ. Surgical issues in the management of carcinoma of the cervix in pregnancy. *Surg Clin North Am* 1995 ; 75 : 89-100

[23] Madej JG Jr. Colposcopy monitoring in pregnancy complicated by CIN and early cervical cancer. *Eur J Gynaecol Oncol* 1996 ; 17 : 59-65

[24] Monk BJ, Montz FJ. Invasive cervical cancer complicating intrauterine pregnancy: Treatment with radical hysterectomy. *Obstet Gynecol* 1992 ; 80 : 199-203

[25] Morris M, Eifel PJ, Lu J, Grigsby PW, Levenback C, Stevens RE et al. Pelvic radiation with concurrent chemotherapy compared with pelvic and para-aortic radiation for high-risk cervical cancer. *N Engl J Med* 1999 ; 340 : 1137-1143

[26] Muñoz N. Human papillomavirus and cervical cancer: epidemiological evidence. In : Franco E, Monsonego J eds. New development in cervical cancer screening and prevention. London : Blackwell Science, 1997 : 3-13

[27] Penna C, Fallani MG, Maggiorelli M, Zipoli E, Cardelli A, Marchionni M. High-grade cervical intraepithelial neoplasia (CIN) in pregnancy: clinicotherapeutic management. *Tumori* 1998 ; 84 : 567-570

[28] Rose PG, Bundy BN, Watkins EB, Thigpen JT, Deppe G, Maiman MA et al. Concurrent cisplatin-based radiotherapy and chemotherapy for locally advanced cervical cancer. *N Engl J Med* 1999 ; 340 : 1144-1153

[29] Sivanesaratnam V, Jayalakshmi P, Loo C. Surgical management of early invasive cancer of the cervix associated with pregnancy. *Gynecol Oncol* 1993 ; 48 : 68-75

[30] Sood AK, Sorosky JI, Krogman S, Anderson B, Benda J, Buller RE. Surgical management of cervical cancer complicating pregnancy: a case control study. *Gynecol Oncol* 1996 ; 63 : 294-298

[31] Sood AK, Sorosky JI, Mayr N, Krogman S, Anderson B, Buller RE et al. Radiotherapeutic management of cervical carcinoma that complicates pregnancy. *Cancer* 1997 ; 80 : 1073-1078

[32] Sorosky JI, Cherouny P, Podczaski ES, Hackett T. Stage IB cervical carcinoma in pregnancy: Awaiting fetal maturity. *J Gynecol Technol* 1996 ; 2 : 155-158

[33] Sorosky JI, Squatrito R, Ndubisi BU, Anderson B, Podczaski ES, Mayr N et al. Stage I squamous cell cervical carcinoma in pregnancy: planned delay in therapy awaiting fetal maturity. *Gynecol Oncol* 1995 ; 59 : 207-210

[34] Subak LL, Hricak H, Powell CB, Azizi L, Stern JL. Cervical carcinoma: computed tomography and magnetic resonance imaging for preoperative staging. *Obstet Gynecol* 1995 ; 86 : 43-50

[35] Tewari K, Cappuccini F, Gambino A, Kohlere MF, Pecorelli S, Disaia PJ. Neoadjuvant chemotherapy in the treatment of locally advanced cervical carcinoma in pregnancy: a report of two cases and review of issues specific to the management of cervical carcinoma in pregnancy including planned delay of therapy. *Cancer* 1998 ; 82 : 1529-1534

[36] Ursin G, Peters RK, Henderson BE, D'Ablaing G 3rd, Monroe KR, Pike MC. Oral contraceptive use and adenocarcinoma of cervix. *Lancet* 1994 ; 344 : 1390-1394

[37] Van Der Vange N, Weverling GJ, Ketting BW, Ankum WM, Samlal R, Lammes FB. The prognosis of cervical cancer associated with pregnancy: a matched cohort study. *Obstet Gynecol* 1995 ; 85 : 1022-1026

[38] Young RH, Scully RE. Villoglandular papillary adenocarcinoma of the uterine cervix. A clinicopathologic analysis of 13 cases. *Cancer* 1989 ; 63 : 1773-1779

[39] Zemlickis D, Lishner M, Degendorfer P, Panzarella T, Sutcliffe SB, Koren G. Maternal and fetal outcome after invasive cervical cancer in pregnancy. *J Clin Oncol* 1991 ; 9 : 1956-1961

[40] Zemlickis D, Lishner M, Degendorfer P, Panzarella T, Sutcliffe SB, Koren G. Fetal outcome after in utero exposure to cancer chemotherapy. *Arch Intern Med* 1992 ; 152 : 573-576

Test yourself – Questions/Answers

Chapter 1 – New concepts in epidemiology of cervical carcinoma

1. *Why are the trends in cervical cancer mortality difficult to interpret?*
    a. Poor quality of death certification.
    b. Different patterns at different ages.
    c. Reduced magnitude of trends.

2. *For which histological type of cervical cancer is the incidence increasing?*
    a. Squamous cell carcinoma.
    b. Adenocarcinoma.
    c. Sarcoma.

3. *In the European Union, which country has the highest incidence rate (after standardisation of the age structure of the world population)?*
    a. Denmark.
    b. Finland.
    c. Portugal.
    d. Spain.

4. *Which of the following are risk factors for cervical cancer?*
    a. Low parity.
    b. Age at menarche.
    c. High number of sexual partners.
    d. Human papilloma virus.

5. *Is smoking a risk factor for cervical cancer?*
    a. Yes.
    b. No.

Answers:
1a,b; 2b; 3c; 4c,d; 5a.

Chapter 2 – Problems in screening of cervical carcinoma

1. *The chances of a CIN I lesion regressing spontaneously and the risk of progression to CIN III are:*
    a. 80% and 10%, respectively.
    b. 57% and 11%, respectively.
    c. 43% and 22%, respectively.
    d. 32% and 30%, respectively.
    e. 55% and 32%, respectively.

2. *The rate of false negative cervical smears is 10-40%. What proportion can be attributed to cell sampling and preparation procedures?*
    a. 1/3.
    b. 1/4.
    c. 1/5.
    d. 3/4.
    e. 1/10.

3. *Before the decision to stop screening women beyond 60 years of age, efforts should be made to identify women who still have an increased risk of developing cervical cancer. They are:*
    a. Women who have participated in the programme but who have a familial history of cervical cancer.
    b. Women using combined hormone replacement therapy.
    c. Women who have had a total hysterectomy due to a benign disease.
    d. Women who have not been correctly screened or have had equivocal smears.
    e. Women who have used oral contraceptives for more than 20 years.

4. *Which one of the following statements is correct?*
    a. Screening 20% of the targeted population every year will reduce the incidence in cervical cancer by less than half of the reduction obtained by screening 80% of the same population every tenth year.
    b. The oncogenic properties of HPV are encoded in the L1-L2 region of the HPV genome.
    c. HPV 16 is the predominant viral subtype associated with cervical adenocarcinoma.
    d. Women with one ASCUS smear can be referred for routine screening intervals if one follow-up smear is normal.
    e. Cytology indicating HPV-NCIN has the same risk of progression to CIN III as CIN I.

5. *Which one of the following statements is incorrect?*
    a. A positive high-risk HPV test predicts high grade SIL more accurately than a repeat smear in women with ASCUS smears.
    b. Liquid-based cytology has higher sensitivity but lower specificity for the presence of high grade SIL than conventional PAP smears.
    c. Liquid-based cytology has higher sensitivity and approximately the same specificity for the presence of high grade SIL as compared to the conventional PAP smear.
    d. Women with HPV-NCIN lesions do not have an increased risk of developing cervical cancer.
    e. Women who have been treated by conisation due to CIN III have an increased risk of developing invasive cervical cancer even after 10 years of follow-up.

Answers:
1b; 2d; 3d; 4a; 5b.

Chapter 3 – Problems in the diagnosis of invasive cervical carcinoma

True or false?

1. *Cervical cancer:*
    a. Is a common cancer in developed countries.
    b. The majority of cervical cancers in developing countries are at an advanced stage at presentation.
    c. A high educational level in women is an important factor in early presentation.
    d. Most cervical cancers are asymptomatic.
    e. The cervical smear is diagnostic for invasive disease in many cases.

2. *Symptoms associated with presentation of cervical cancer are:*
    a. Offensive vaginal discharge.
    b. Backache.
    c. Weight gain.
    d. Postmenopausal bleeding.
    e. Early menopause.

3. *Colposcopic features of invasive cervical cancer are:*
    a. Atrophic cervix.
    b. Atypical vessels.
    c. Contact bleeding.
    d. Smooth surface.
    e. Ulcerated lesions.

4. *Diagnostic techniques for cervical carcinoma are:*
    a. Colposcopy alone.
    b. Punch biopsy is usually adequate.
    c. Endocervical curettage is mandatory.
    d. Knife cone biopsy.
    e. Diathermy excision of transformation zone.

5. *Cervical carcinoma in pregnancy:*
    a. 10% of cervical cancers are diagnosed during pregnancy.
    b. Visual inspection of the cervix is important if there is bleeding during pregnancy.
    c. Outpatient biopsy is a safe diagnostic test to confirm invasive disease.
    d. The changes in pregnancy can be difficult to assess.
    e. A biopsy should be undertaken whenever there is any uncertainty with colposcopy.

Answers:
1. a.false; b.true; c.true; d.false; e.false.
2. a.true; b.true; c.false; d.true; e.false.
3. a.false; b.true; c.true; d.false; e.true.
4. a.false; b.false; c.false; d.true; e.true.
5. a.false; b.true; c.false; d.true; e.false.

Chapter 4 – Pathology of cervical carcinoma

1. *All of the following statements concerning adenocarcinoma are correct except one. Identify it.*
    a. The great majority of cervical adenocarcinomas are primitive endocervical neoplasia.
    b. Endometroid carcinoma is a common type of primitive endocervical neoplasia.
    c. Serous carcinoma is very aggressive even with minimal infiltration.
    d. Clear cell carcinoma can occur in older patients without any history of DES exposition.
    e. The incidence of adenocarcinoma is increasing, notably in young women.

2. *All of the following statements concerning micro-invasive carcinoma are correct except one. Identify it.*
    a. Infiltration is limited to 5 mm below the stratified lining.
    b. No vascular invasion is present.
    c. It can develop from a gland colonised by CIN.
    d. Conservative treatment is justified as with CIN.
    e. It has no metastatic potential.

3. *All of the following statements concerning squamous cell carcinoma are correct except one. Identify it.*
    a. Verrucous carcinoma should not be treated with radiotherapy.
    b. Infiltration could be difficult to visualise in biopsies from papillary or warty carcinomas.
    c. Squamous cell carcinoma is the more common type of cervical carcinoma.
    d. Squamous cell carcinoma does not always develop from a CIN nor is it always related to HPV infection.
    e. Histological grading reliably predicts prognosis.

4. *All of the following statements concerning these neoplasia are correct except one. Identify it.*
    a. Adenoid basal carcinoma can be an incidental finding without any metastatic potential.
    b. Adenoid cystic carcinoma can be deeply invasive with a worse prognosis.
    c. Glassy cell carcinoma is a variant of adenocarcinoma or adenosquamous carcinoma.
    d. Among neuroendocrinal tumours, true primary carcinoid tumours of the cervix can be observed.
    e. Metastatic carcinomas of the cervix are a rather rare event.

5. *All of the following statements concerning cervical carcinomas are correct except one. Identify it.*
    a. Adenocarcinoma and CIN can be associated and related to the presence of HPV infestation.
    b. The concept of micro-invasive carcinoma is as well defined for adenocarcinoma as for squamous cell carcinoma.
    c. The general extension or spread of adenocarcinoma and squamous cell carcinoma is somewhat similar.
    d. Neuroendocrine differentiation can occur in several types of adenocarcinoma.
    e. In the cervix, metastatic carcinomas can simulate a primitive carcinoma both clinically and morphologically.

Answers:
1a; 2a; 3e; 4d; 5b.

Chapter 5 – Staging and pretherapeutic investigations

1. *All the following statements concerning cervical cancer staging are correct except one. Identify it.*
   a. Staging allows the comparison of results from different institutions.
   b. The great majority of patients with cervical cancer will have a normal general physical examination.
   c. Clinical examination under anaesthesia should be performed.
   d. Staging can be changed according to the findings at surgery.
   e. Staging does not limit the therapeutic strategies.

2. *The only colposcopic finding mentioned below that is suggestive of early cervical cancer is:*
   a. Acetowhite epithelium.
   b. Mosaic.
   c. Punctation.
   d. Both mosaic and punctation.
   e. Abnormal blood vessels.

3. *Concerning the clinical staging of cervical carcinoma, choose the true statement.*
   a. Stage Ia1 corresponds to lesions with less than 3 mm invasion.
   b. Vascular space involvement is independent of the depth of invasion only in stage Ia.
   c. A cancer strictly confined to the cervix with more than 3 cm in diameter should be allotted to stage Ib2.
   d. When there is doubt concerning the stage to which a cancer should be assigned, the earlier stage should be chosen.
   e. The presence of hydronephrosis and non-functioning kidney always allows a tumour to be assigned to stage IIIb.

4. *Only one of the following studies is optional for the staging of cervical cancer. Identify it.*
   a. Chest X-ray.
   b. Rectosigmoidoscopy.
   c. Computerised axial tomography.
   d. Cystoscopy.
   e. Skeletal X-ray.

5. *All the following assertions are correct except:*
   a. CT scan allows effective visualisation of the thorax and upper abdomen.
   b. CT scan permits the study of the bowel after contrast medium has been used.
   c. MRI-guided fine-needle aspiration biopsy is effective to study the nature of a suspect pelvic mass.
   d. MRI has a greater capacity than CT scan in discriminating between cancer and normal cervical tissue.
   e. MRI is superior to CT scan in evaluating the parametrial extension of a cervical tumour.

Answers:
1d; 2e; 3d; 4c; 5c.

Chapter 6 – Treatment of micro-invasive cervical carcinoma

1. *Is there evidence that simple hysterectomy is superior to conisation in controlling squamous cell microcarcinoma localised in the uterine cervix?*
   a. Hysterectomy is superior to conisation.
   b. Adequate conisation is equally effective.
   c. Hysterectomy is superior to conisation in postmenopausal but not in premenopausal women.
   d. Conisation is not so effective if the disease is multifocal.

2. *Is there a place for lymphadenectomy in stage IA1 squamous cervical carcinoma?*
   a. Yes, because the incidence of pelvic lymph node involvement is substantial.
   b. Only in the presence of LVSI.
   c. No, because the risk of pelvic node metastasis is negligible.
   d. Only if the margins are positive.

3. *If the cone biopsy margin is not clear, should a simple hysterectomy be performed?*
   a. No, a repeat cone excision is required after wound healing - about 6 weeks postoperatively - to rule out higher stage disease.
   b. Yes, to be sure the lesion is completely excised.
   c. Yes, because in the presence of positive margins the disease is often multifocal.
   d. Only if there is no concern of further childbearing.

4. *Does parametrial excision improve outcome?*
   a. Only in stage IA2 lesions.
   b. There is no convincing evidence to support this approach.
   c. Only in the presence of LVSI.
   d. Yes, in the presence of residual disease in the hysterectomy specimen.

5. *Is conisation an adequate treatment for micro-adenocarcinoma?*
   a. Yes, there is no evidence that simple hysterectomy is superior.
   b. Only if the lymph nodes are negative.
   c. Yes, provided the excision margins are free of disease.
   d. No, because residual disease is frequent in the hysterectomy specimen even when the surgical margins are negative.

Answers:
1b; 2c; 3a; 4b; 5d.

Chapter 7 – Radical abdominal hysterectomy for stage I and II cervical carcinoma

1. *Which anatomical structures are removed at radical abdominal hysterectomy?*
   a. The uterus with parametrium, vaginal cuff with paracolpos and the pelvic lymph nodes.
   b. The uterus, tubes and ovaries and pelvic lymph nodes.
   c. The uterus, omentum, pelvic and paraaortic lymph nodes and intra-abdominal disease.

2. *What are the anatomical borders of the paravesical and pararectal spaces?*
   a. Peritoneum, broad ligament and symphysis.
   b. Infundibulopelvic ligament, broad ligament and cardinal ligament.
   c. Obliterated umbilical artery and lateral aspect of the urinary bladder, posterior aspect of the symphysis and pubic part of the levator ani muscle, external iliac vessels and medial aspect of the internal oblique muscle and the anterior aspect of the lateral parametrium and paracolpos.

3. *Name two significant prognostic factors in patients with surgically treated cervical cancer.*
   a. Lymph node status and tumour size.
   b. Histological grade and tumour size.
   c. Ploidy and parametrial extension.

4. *Is salpingo-oophorectomy indicated in premenopausal women with stage IB to IIB cervical cancer undergoing radical hysterectomy?*
   a. Yes.
   b. No.

5. *What are the most common complications of radical hysterectomy?*
   a. Thromboembolic disease.
   b. Urinary tract infection.
   c. Voiding dysfunction.

———————

Answers:
1a; 2c; 3a; 4b; 5c.

Chapter 8 – Radiotherapy for stage I-II cervical cancer

1. *Geographical missing of macroscopic disease by external beam radiation therapy to the pelvis for cervical cancer most frequently occurs at:*
 a. The inferior border of the AP-PA fields.
 b. The anterior border of the lateral fields.
 c. The superior border of the lateral fields.
 d. The posterior border of the lateral fields.
 e. The lateral border of the AP-PA fields.

2. *When delivering 75 Gy to Point A with uterovaginal brachytherapy (including external beam radiotherapy doses and assuming an identical source geometry of the brachytherapy), the highest bladder and rectal doses will be delivered by:*
 a. Brachytherapy alone (75 Gy to Point A).
 b. 50 Gy EBRT and BT (in total, 75 Gy to Point A).
 c. EBRT (with partial shielding by central block in the anteroposterior fields) to 50 Gy and BT (in total, 75 Gy to Point A).
 d. It makes no difference.

3. *When treating a patient with cervical cancer by radical radiotherapy and HDR brachytherapy with a total duration of 7 weeks instead of 9 weeks:*
 a. Results will be worse because complication rates will increase dramatically (15-20% grade 2-3).
 b. Survival will be improved by 4 to 11%.
 c. Local control will be improved by 15 to 22%, without impact on survival.
 d. Local control will be improved by 11 to 15%, but the impact on survival is partially cancelled by lethal complications.
 e. Treatment outcome is not affected by the difference in duration of the treatment.

4. *In a multivariate assessment, which of the following factors least affects local control after radical radiotherapy?*
 a. Haemoglobin level more or less than 12g/L.
 b. Stage Ib versus stage IIa, IIb.
 c. Tumour size greater or smaller than 6 cm.
 d. Adenocarcinoma versus squamous cell carcinoma.

_____
Answers:
1d; 2b; 3b; 4c,d.

Chapter 9 – Radiation therapy and surgical treatment of cervical carcinoma stages IB and II

1. *What is the conventional treatment for carcinoma of the cervix when the lesion is 30 mm in diameter with histological evidence of pelvic lymph node involvement?*
    a. External irradiation – colpohysterectomy with lymphadenectomy – vaginal curietherapy.
    b. Combined radiotherapy and chemotherapy - colpohysterectomy with lymphadenectomy – vaginal curietherapy.
    c. Uterovaginal curietherapy – colpohysterectomy with lymphadenectomy – external irradiation.
    d. Colpohysterectomy with lymphadenectomy – external irradiation – utero-vaginal curietherapy.

2. *Survival rates after treatment by surgery alone, by radiotherapy associated with surgery, or by radiotherapy alone are:*
    a. Higher after surgery alone.
    b. Higher after radiotherapy combined with surgery.
    c. Higher after radiotherapy alone.
    d. Comparable for all three.

3. *Of the following, which apply to preoperative curietherapy for small cervical cancers (< 40 mm)?*
    a. Regression, or better, sterilisation of the cervix is a good prognosis factor.
    b. The presence of the uterus allows central pelvic irradiation under optimal conditions.
    c. Curietherapy allows pelvic irradiation including the lymph nodes.
    d. Curietherapy reduces the extent of surgery.

4. *Concering a proximal colpohysterectomy, which of the following are true?*
    a. It always allows preservation of the ovaries due to the low incidence of ovarian metastases.
    b. The entire uterus and vaginal collar are surgically removed.
    c. At the parametrial level, excision passes outside the ureters and the external pillars of the bladder.
    d. It is associated with lymphadenectomy (pelvic and possibly para-aortic).

5. *Among the following complications, which is the most frequent after both surgery and radiotherapy?*
    a. Pelvic lymphoceles.
    b. Lower limb lymphoedema.
    c. Digestive stenosis.
    d. Ureteral stenosis.

Answers:
1c; 2d; 3a,b,d; 4b,d; 5b.

Chapter 10 – Laparoscopic approach: new concepts of treatment of cervical carcinoma stages I and II

1. A patient presents with a stage IB1 squamous cell carcinoma of the cervix. A laparoscopic interiliac node dissection is performed; no metastasis is found at frozen section examination. The probability of involvement of common iliac or aortic nodes is:
  a. Less than 1%.
  b. 2%.
  c. 4%.
  d. 8%.
  e. 10%.

2. The surgical term "interiliac lymphadenectomy" means which following node groups are removed?
  a. Nodes located between the external iliac artery and the external iliac vein.
  b. Nodes located between the common iliac artery and the common iliac vein.
  c. Nodes located between the branches of bifurcation of the common iliac artery.
  d. Nodes located between the right and left common iliac artery.
  e. Nodes located in the distal part of the cardinal ligament.

3. A laparoscopically assisted, modified radical vaginal hysterectomy is adequate as definitive therapy for:
  a. Stage IA2 cervical cancers only.
  b. Stage IA2 and stage IB1 less than 2 cm in diameter.
  c. Stage IA2 and IB1.
  d. Stage IA2, IB1 and IB2.
  e. Stage I and II.

4. In carcinomas of the cervix IB-II with negative iliac nodes, the probability of involvement of the paracervical nodes is:
  a. 0%.
  b. 2%.
  c. 5%.
  d. 10%.
  e. 20%.

5. The extraperitoneal endoscopic approach using the left lower quadrant is adequate for removing:
  a. Inframesenteric lateroaortic nodes only.
  b. Inframesenteric and infrarenal lateroaortic nodes only.
  c. Inframesenteric aortic and common iliac nodes only.
  d. Inframesenteric and infrarenal aortic nodes along with common iliac nodes.
  e. Obturator, common iliac, and aortic nodes on the left side only.

Answers:
1a; 2c; 3b; 4c; 5d.

Chapter 11 – Bulky stage I and II cervical carcinoma: a therapeutic dilemma

True or false?

1. *Concerning lymph node metastases:*
   a. The incidence increases with increasing diameter of the primary tumour.
   b. When the common iliac nodes are positive, the 5-year survival is approximately 25%.
   c. 50 Gy of external beam radiotherapy will eradicate 90% of 2 cm nodes.
   d. Bilateral positive pelvic lymph nodes have a worse prognosis (22-40% 5-year survival) than unilateral positive pelvic nodes (59-70%).
   e. Surgical removal of bulky lymph nodes may improve 5-year survival.

2. *Concerning radical radiotherapy for primary cervical carcinoma:*
   a. It is given over a period of three weeks.
   b. After brachytherapy, the radiation dose reaches a total of 80-90 Gy at point A.
   c. It has inferior overall cure rates compared to surgery.
   d. It can produce haematological side effects.
   e. It may be less effective than surgery in bulky adenocarcinoma of the cervix.

3. *Concurrent chemoradiotherapy:*
   a. Improves survival in bulky cervical tumours compared to radiation alone.
   b. Hydroxyurea has been shown to be the most effective drug in concurrent chemoradiotherapy.
   c. The chemotherapy acts as a radiosensitiser.
   d. Increases the haematological side effects compared to radiation alone.
   e. Reduces pelvic recurrences when compared to radiation alone.

4. *Surgical staging:*
   a. Is no more accurate than clinical staging.
   b. Lymphograms are a sensitive and specific method of detecting nodal metastases.
   c. Can be undertaken laparoscopically.
   d. Can be used to plan radiation fields.
   e. May allow salvage of women with nodal metastases outside the pelvis that can be treated with extended field radiotherapy.

5. *Prognostic factors for survival in women with cervical carcinoma are:*
   a. The status of the lymph nodes.
   b. The size of the tumour.
   c. Involvement of paracervical tissues.
   d. Depth of invasion.
   e. The presence of lymphovascular invasion.

_____

Answers:
1. a.true; b.true; c.false; d.true; e.true.
2. a.false; b.true; c.false; d.true; e.true.
3. a.true; b.false; c.true; d.true; e.true.
4. a.false; b.false; c.true; d.true; e.true.
5. a.true; b.true; c.true; d.true; e.true.

Chapter 12 – Treatment of cervical carcinoma stages III and IV

1. *Cervical carcinoma is diagnosed at stage III-IV in about:*
   a. 5%.
   b. 15%.
   c. 25%.
   d. 45% of cases.

2. *Standard treatment for stage III-IVA patients is:*
   a. Preoperative chemotherapy followed by surgery.
   b. Exclusive radiotherapy.
   c. Concurrent chemotherapy and radiotherapy.
   d. Palliative therapies.

3. *Curative radiotherapy for stage III-IVA patients consists of:*
   a. External beam RT.
   b. External beam RT followed by brachytherapy.
   c. Brachytherapy followed by external beam RT.
   d. Brachytherapy.

4. *The drug of choice for concurrent chemotherapy and radiation in cervical carcinoma is:*
   a. Cisplatin.
   b. Hydroxyurea.
   c. Carboplatin.
   d. 5-FU and hydroxyurea.

5. *In naive patients with cervical carcinoma at stage III, the clinical response rate following preoperative chemotherapy is about:*
   a. 15-20%.
   b. 30-40%.
   c. 50-60%.
   d. 70-80%.

Answers:
1c; 2b; 3b; 4a; 5d.

Chapter 13 – Recurrence of cervical carcinoma: risk factors and treatment

1. *Which of the following risk factors is the least important when considering the planning of primary treatment?*
   a. The FIGO stage.
   b. Nodal involvement.
   c. Size of the tumour.
   d. Histological type.

2. *Which of the following statements concerning recurrences of cervical cancer is not true?*
   a. Following surgery alone, most of the recurrences (60-70%) will be located within the pelvis.
   b. Following radiation therapy, most of the recurrences will be at distant (extrapelvic) sites.
   c. Prognosis of recurrent cervical cancer depends mainly on location and primary treatment.
   d. Early recurrences (within 6 months after primary treatment) have a higher chance of cure.

3. *Which of the following examinations should be routinely carried out during the follow-up of patients with cervical cancer?*
   a. Clinical evaluation and cytology.
   b. Chest X-rays, IVP and abdominal u/s.
   c. CT and MRI of the abdomen.
   d. All of the above.

4. *Which of the following statements concerning the management of recurrent cervical cancer is not correct?*
   a. Central pelvic recurrences after radiation therapy are best treated with aggressive surgery.
   b. Central pelvic recurrences after surgery alone should be considered for radiation therapy.
   c. Recurrent tumour involving the pelvic side-wall following radiation therapy is best treated by chemotherapy only.

5. *Which of the following factors is regarded as a contraindication to exenterative surgery?*
   a. The presence of distant site metastasis.
   b. Para-aortic node involvement.
   c. Patient with poor surgical risk.
   d. All of the above.

Answers:
1d; 2d; 3a; 4c; 5d.

Chapter 14 – Management of early cervical carcinoma associated with pregnancy

1. *Please mark the correct answer regarding cervical carcinoma complicating pregnancy:*
    a. It is a relatively common association.
    b. It is more common in the fourth decade of life.
    c. The prevalence of human papilloma virus (HPV) DNA in these patients is up to 100% in some series.
    d. Adenocarcinoma is the most frequent histological type.
    e. Pain is the earliest clinical symptom.

2. *A 29-year-old primigravida in her twenty-first week of gestation presented to the hospital because of occasional vaginal bleeding following coitus. An obstetric ultrasound study did not reveal placental abnormalities. The diagnostic attitude is:*
    a. Perform a magnetic resonance imaging (MRI) study.
    b. Anamnesis, gynaecological examination and cervicovaginal cytology.
    c. Rectosigmoidoscopy.
    d. Tocolytic drugs and wait for the response.
    e. Order a haemogram to assess blood coagulation defects.

3. *In respect to performing a conisation during pregnancy, which answer is incorrect?*
    a. It should be performed when colposcopic examination is unsuccessful.
    b. It should be performed when colposcopic findings are not consistent with cytological abnormalities.
    c. It should be performed in case of suspicion of micro-invasive carcinoma.
    d. It should always be performed in low-grade squamous intraepithelial lesions.
    e. Cervical conisation is advisable when biopsy shows an adenocarcinoma.

4. *Indicate the correct answer regarding treatment of cervical carcinoma associated with pregnancy.*
    a. FIGO staging of carcinoma of the cervix is not relevant as a prognostic factor.
    b. Treatment modality of choice should never be delayed by gestational age at the time of diagnosis.
    c. Therapeutic options for pregnant women are similar to those for their non-pregnant counterparts.
    d. The course of pregnancy is always associated with a progression of the cervical lesion.
    e. Radical surgery should not be carried out immediately following a caesarean section.

5. *A colposcopic-guided biopsy in a pregnant woman in her thirty-fourth week of gestation suggests a micro-invasive carcinoma. Cervical conisation shows stage IA1 squamous cell carcinoma with no lymph-vascular space invasion. The margins of the cone are negative. The most adequate attitude is:*

 a. Termination of pregnancy by caesarean section followed by radical hysterectomy and pelvic lymph-node dissection.

 b. Spontaneous vaginal delivery and evaluation of a subsequent total hysterectomy according to future child-bearing expectations.

 c. Immediate caesarean section followed by endocavitary radiation therapy.

 d. Neoadjuvant chemotherapy and surgical treatment once pregnancy has been terminated.

 e. No follow-up at all after delivery.

Answers:
1c; 2b; 3d; 4c; 5b.

Index